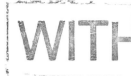

D0866091

Contents

About the authors

Kath Sharples is Director of Practice and Work-based Learning at the University of West London. As an experienced registered nurse and registered nurse teacher, Kath has a comprehensive understanding of the current challenges and developments within nurse education. Her main area of pedagogic interest and research activity is related to self-regulated learning in practice. Kath's expertise is in preparing students for practice learning and developing mentors in their responsibility as gatekeepers to the profession.

Karen Elcock is Head of Programmes, Pre-registration Nursing, at the Faculty of Health and Social Care Sciences, Kingston University and St George's University in London. Her professional interests lie in practice education, with particular focus on how students are prepared for learning in practice, mentor development and support and the development of support roles to practice.

Acknowledgements

The authors and publisher wish to thank the following for permission to reproduce copyright material:

Gibb's Reflective Model (Figure 3.1), taken from Gibbs, G (1988) *Learning and Doing: A Guide to Teaching and Learning Methods*. Oxford: Further Education Unit, Oxford Polytechnic, and reproduced by kind permission of Oxford Brookes University.

Honey and Mumford Learning Styles quoted on pages 19–20, taken from Honey, P and Mumford, A (1992) *The Manual of Learning Styles*. Maidenhead: Peter Honey Publications, and reproduced by kind permission of EDI Ltd.

The Thomas–Kilmann conflict management styles (Figure 11.1) is taken from Thomas, K (1992) Conflict and Negotiation Process in Organizations, in MD Dunnette and LM Hough (eds) *Handbook of Industrial and Organizational Psychology*, 2nd edn, vol. 3, page 660. Palo Alto, CA: Consulting Psychologists Press, © 1992 LM Hough, adapted with permission, and reproduced by kind permission of Consulting Psychologists Press Inc.

Standing's revised cognitive continuum of clinical judgement and decision-making in nursing (Figure 15.1) is taken from Standing, M (2008) Clinical judgement and decision-making in nursing – nine modes of practice in a revised cognitive continuum, *Journal of Advanced Nursing*, 62(1): 130, by kind permission of John Wiley and Sons.

Dedication

Karen: to Steve, for all your support and encouragement. I know how proud you would have been.

Kath: to Ann, for putting up with my tapping (again).

Introduction

Who is this book for?

This book has been written primarily for newly registered nurses who are undertaking their first post following completion of a pre-registration nursing programme. The first year post qualification is both exciting and daunting in equal measure. There will be expectations of you, and expectations by you, that provide numerous opportunities and challenges in terms of your professional development. This book is intended to aid new registrants as they embrace the challenges of undertaking a preceptorship programme. Rather than replace preceptorship programmes, the contents of the book are intended to provide 'added value' to the various elements of your preceptorship programme, helping you as a newly registered nurse to explore some of the challenges and opportunities you may encounter during the transition period from student to accountable practitioner.

Additionally, this book will be of value to nursing students who are approaching the final stages of their pre-registration programme and are moving towards their first post as registered nurses.

Book structure

Chapter 1, Beginning the preceptorship journey, provides a context to the preceptorship framework and explains its relationship to the knowledge and skills framework. The chapter will assist you to contextualise the key elements of the preceptorship framework while reflecting on how the knowledge and skills framework is relevant to you and your career. In addition, the chapter will help you to identify the key elements of the preceptor role and develop an appreciation of your responsibilities as a newly registered nurse.

Chapter 2, Developing confidence and self-awareness, will assist you to identify specific learning and professional development needs that will underpin your preceptorship programme. The chapter will guide you in the principles of undertaking a self-assessment of your learning needs and current learning style. You will be able to use this knowledge to implement adult learning strategies and promote future self-awareness of your developmental needs.

Chapter 3, Reflection and receiving feedback, allows you to explore the use of reflection and feedback to support your professional development. The chapter allows you to select the model of reflection that may be most appropriate for you to use in a practice setting. By the end of the chapter you will have gained confidence in seeking and receiving feedback on your performance in practice and be able to identify links between self-awareness and reflection in relation to professional development.

Chapter 4, Integrating prior learning into practice, provides a platform for you to identify specific learning and professional development needs based on the outcome of reflection and feedback. In reading the chapter and participating in the activities provided you will be able to clarify specific learning needs and also develop learning plans that support your professional development needs. In addition, you will be able to identify both current and future opportunities for utilising experiential learning within your practice area.

Chapter 5, Increasing knowledge and clinical skills, assists you to recognise the value of professional development opportunities in relation to formal and informal assessment and staff-development events. The chapter also includes a variety of practical advice related to preparation for competency testing and using an experiential model to achieve your development goals. You will also gain insight into the purpose of peer review/clinical supervision.

Chapter 6, Confidence in applying evidence-based practice, considers the role of the registered nurse in relation to identifying and implementing evidence-based practice. Not only will you be able to revisit the importance of applying research to nursing practice but you will also be able to identify strategies for implementing evidence-based practice. The chapter also explores practical ways to keep you up to date.

Chapter 7, Understanding policies and procedures, provides an opportunity to explore the importance of understanding policies and procedures and your own accountability and responsibility in relation to them. In reading this chapter you will be able to appreciate your own responsibility and accountability with regard to implementing and following policies and procedures. In addition, you will also develop an understanding of how policies are developed both within your current organisation and nationally, and how to access them.

Chapter 8, Team-working, assists you to investigate your role within the multidisciplinary team. You will develop a clear appreciation of why teamwork is essential in healthcare and your current role and responsibilities within the team. In so doing you will also identify the key members of the multidisciplinary teams you work with, gain insight into the challenges of team-working and develop strategies to manage these challenges.

Chapter 9, Communication and interpersonal skills, promotes strategies for developing your interpersonal skills. There is advice on implementing a range of practical communication strategies, such as understanding professional communication strategies when using email as a communication tool. You will also gain insight into the range of communication strategies that will be required within your professional role, exploring practical techniques for improving your written/verbal communication and maintaining accurate records.

Chapter 10, Advocacy, is intended to further your understanding of the nurse's role as an advocate, including professional implications for advocacy in practice. You will be able to identify your advocacy role as a member of the multidisciplinary team and recognise the attributes of assertiveness as opposed to aggression. The chapter also promotes an understanding of the implications of advocacy in relation to the NMC Code of Conduct.

Chapter 11, Negotiation and conflict resolution, identifies the various ways that conflict may arise within the nursing environment. Specifically, the chapter looks at how the skills of negotiation and conflict resolution can be used to prevent the negative consequences that can arise where conflict is not resolved. In so doing you will be able to identify the common causes of conflict within the practice setting and appreciate the impact of conflict on people and the work environment.

There is also practical advice in terms of managing conflict, patient complaints and the steps that can be taken to reduce the likelihood of complaints. In addition, there is advice provided on the steps that should be taken when responding to patient complaints.

Chapter 12, Implementing the Code and professional values, allows you to investigate professionalism and accountability as a newly registered nurse. This will involve reflection on the implications for you in becoming a registered nurse and an appreciation of the importance of demonstrating professional behaviour. You will also have an opportunity to reflect on your professional values, explain the difference between responsibility and accountability and in so doing explain the different types of accountability and their relevance to yourself.

Chapter 13, Managing risk, explores the major elements of risk assessment and assists you in developing an understanding of implementing risk assessment and management tools within practice. You will revisit the key policies associated with risk assessment and management within the NHS and recognise the value of clinical governance and audit in identifying and preventing clinical risk. The chapter provides insight into the relationship between professional responsibility and risk by exploring incident reporting and 'whistleblowing' in relation to risk management.

Chapter 14, Equality and diversity, assists you to gain a fresh understanding of equality and diversity issues within healthcare and how these relate to your professional role. The chapter identifies the key elements of equality and diversity and explores the principles for managing these issues within an organisation. You will be able to draw links between equality and diversity in relation to care of patients and your membership within an organisation.

Chapter 15, Decision-making, helps you to understand decision-making in the context of clinical practice. You will be able to consider different approaches to problem-solving and decision-making and identify the sources of information or knowledge that you can use to help you make decisions. These factors will aid you to appreciate the importance of shared decision-making and the nurse's role in supporting patients through the decision-making process.

Chapter 16, Leadership and management development, explores your role as a leader within a team. You will begin the chapter by identifying the skills required for managing and leading care and then considering the strategies you can use to lead a team effectively. Your responsibilities with regard to delegation and appreciating the implications in delegating care activities will be discussed so you may understand your role and responsibilities in supporting learners.

Chapter 17, Developing an outcome approach to continuing professional development, will assist you in considering how you will plan your ongoing professional development. You will initially reflect on how the Knowledge and Skills Framework is relevant to you and your career, appreciating the importance of lifelong learning to your professional role. The chapter will provide an opportunity to outline key changes and policy that will influence your future roles and in so doing develop a personal and professional development plan.

Learning features

This book provides a number of activities throughout each chapter that will aid you to understand the issues being discussed. Some of the activities will involve an element of active participation where you may need to look up an additional resource; other activities require you to stop and think about a situation or your reaction to a past experience.

Reflective activities allow you to understand your current context by reviewing a past situation or experience. Critical thinking activities encourage you to challenge your practice to ensure 'best practice' rather than a reliance on tradition. Evidence-based practice activities help you to explore current research and ensure that you are able to defend your role and responsibility as a professional. Decision-making activities allow you to practise this essential skill and identify areas where you may need to further your confidence or knowledge base.

Communication activities also offer practical opportunities for developing your knowledge and skills, and often require you to review your practice with other healthcare professionals. Team-working and leadership activities promote your understanding of your current role within the organisation and can help you to identify future developmental opportunities.

In addition, the book provides 'added value' activities by providing links at the end of each chapter to Flying Start NHS (Scotland), www.flyingstart.scot.nhs.uk, and Flying Start England, www. flyingstartengland.nhs.uk/. Both of these websites provide online development programmes for all newly registered nurses in Scotland and England. The activities recommended to you have been selected as they will support and extend your professional development throughout your preceptorship programme.

The Preceptorship Framework

The *Preceptorship Framework for Newly Registered Nurses, Midwives and Allied Health Professionals* was published in March 2010 and can be found on the Department of Health website (**www.doh. gov.uk**). It is a best practice guidance document that employers both inside and outside the NHS in England may choose to guide the content and structure of preceptorship programmes. Scotland has its own web-based multiprofessional preceptorship programme called Flying Start NHS, which is similar to the Department of Health framework. Likewise, the Welsh and Northern Ireland Assemblies both support the use of preceptorship for new registrants during their first year, although they have not adopted a specific framework as yet. We have therefore decided to utilise the suggested content for preceptorship programmes described in the framework by the Department of Health (2010a) as the basis for the chapters within this book.

Your first year as a registered nurse is an exciting time when you can truly celebrate your achievement. You have worked very hard to achieve your qualification and throughout your career you will be constantly rewarded for your effort and perseverance. However, your first year as a registered nurse will be daunting at times and you will experience a degree of culture shock as you grow into your professional role. The authors of this book acknowledge that you will face a variety of challenges during your first year and we hope that this book supports you as you embark on this exciting journey as a registered nurse. We take this opportunity to wish you every success as you continue throughout your career as a lifelong learner.

Chapter 1
Beginning the preceptorship journey

Preceptorship Framework and KSF

This chapter maps to the following elements of the Department of Health Preceptorship Framework and the NHS Knowledge and Skills Framework.

Preceptorship Framework

- Develop confidence and self-awareness
- Increase knowledge and clinical skills
- Integrate prior learning into practice

NHS Knowledge and Skills Framework

- Communication
- Personal and people development

Chapter aims

The aim of this chapter is to introduce you to the Preceptorship Framework and its relationship to the Knowledge and Skills Framework. By the end of this chapter you will be able to:

- outline the key elements of the Preceptorship Framework;
- explore the benefits of undertaking a preceptorship programme;
- reflect on how the Knowledge and Skills Framework is relevant to you and your career;
- identify the key elements of the preceptor role;
- appreciate your responsibilities as a newly registered nurse.

Setting the scene

Your first day at work as a registered nurse is probably one of the most exciting and nerve wracking days you will encounter. Even if your first post is somewhere you worked as a student, entering that practice area as a qualified nurse will be very different. The challenges of the transition phase from student to staff nurse are well documented in the literature and it was Kramer (1974) who coined the phrase *reality shock* to describe the initial work experience of newly qualified nurses and described the discrepancies that arise between their expectations and the real world of nursing.

If you have just completed a return to practice course or overseas nursing programme, it is likely that you will still have a certain degree of nervousness as you move from your protected role as student to registered nurse.

It is to be hoped that you have found a first post with an employer who runs a preceptorship programme which will help you with this transition. However, this book will help support your first few months as a registered nurse with or without a preceptorship programme in place.

Activity 1.1: Reflection

Identifying your fears

Note down the fears, worries or concerns you had before taking up your first post or in your first few weeks in post.

There is a brief outline answer to this activity at the end of the chapter.

It is not surprising to find that the majority of newly registered nurses want a post where preceptorship is offered (Robinson and Griffiths, 2009) and as a consequence will tend to apply for their first post in the NHS which will provide a structured programme of support for newly qualified practitioners, although increasingly independent sector organisations are recognising the need to offer preceptorship programmes as well.

The need to provide support to newly registered nurses through preceptorship is well recognised (UKCC, 1986, 1993, 1999; Department of Health, 2001a) but it has never been made a mandatory requirement, although Agenda for Change (AfC), the NHS national pay and grading system which was introduced in 2004, identified the need for preceptorship and linked this with the first year for staff in Band 5 posts (The NHS Staff Council, 2010). In 2006 the NMC strongly recommended that all *new registrants have a period of preceptorship of at least four months on commencing employment* (NMC, 2006) and went further as part of its consultation of pre-registration nursing education in 2008 in proposing that there should be a mandatory period of preceptorship for all new registrants. They stepped back, however, from this requirement when they published their *Standards for Pre-registration Nursing Education* (NMC, 2010a) and simply stated that *newly qualified nurses cannot be expected to have extensive clinical experience, specialist expertise, or highly developed supervision and leadership skills* (NMC, 2010a, page 5) and that these skills would be further developed through the preceptorship period and ongoing professional development.

The review of the NHS undertaken by Lord Darzi in 2008 (Department of Health, 2008a) also identified the need for a foundation period of preceptorship for newly qualified nurses, which led to increased funding to support the implementation of preceptorship schemes within the NHS.

All of the above culminated in the publication of the *Preceptorship Framework for Newly Registered Nurses, Midwives and Allied Health Professionals* (Department of Health, 2010a) that could be used as a resource by both employers and newly qualified healthcare professionals in setting and running preceptorship programmes.

What is preceptorship?

There are a number of different definitions for preceptorship, but the one agreed in the Preceptorship Framework is:

A period of structured transition for the newly registered practitioner during which he or she will be supported by a preceptor, to develop their confidence as an autonomous professional, refine skills, values and behaviours and to continue on their journey of life-long learning.
(Department of Health, 2010a, page 11)

Just to confuse matters, many countries outside the UK use the term preceptorship to describe the support provided to student nurses by qualified practitioners which we call mentorship, so care should be taken in reading books or articles on preceptorship as they may not be appropriate to your needs.

Preceptorship in the UK is recommended for all new registrants and that includes:

- newly qualified practitioners registering with the NMC for the first time;
- qualified practitioners registering on a new part of the NMC register having undertaken a further registerable qualification;
- practitioners who have qualified overseas and are newly registered with the NMC;
- practitioners who have completed a return to practice programme and have re-registered with the NMC.

The benefits of preceptorship

As well as easing the transition for newly registered nurses, preceptorship is also perceived as having a number of other potential benefits to the preceptee as well as benefits for the preceptor, the employer and the healthcare professions as a whole (Department of Health, 2010a; Higgens et al., 2010; Roxburgh et al., 2010) including:

- enhanced recruitment;
- improved retention;
- reduced sickness/absence;
- reduction in near-miss incidents made by newly registered nurses;
- personal and professional development for the preceptor in developing appraisal, mentoring, supervising and supportive skills;
- increased confidence and competence for the newly registered nurse.

Central, however, to a preceptorship programme is the drive to ensure that patients/clients and service users receive safe and effective care and treatment and a better patient experience.

Activity 1.2: Reflection

The benefits of preceptorship
Make a list of what you hope to gain from undertaking a preceptorship programme. What are your expectations?

There is a brief outline answer to this activity at the end of the chapter.

The Preceptorship Framework

The *Preceptorship Framework for Newly Registered Nurses, Midwives and Allied Health Professionals* was published in March 2010 and can be found on the Department of Health website (**www.doh. gov.uk**). It is a best-practice guidance document which you can use as a resource but is also useful for employers both inside and outside the NHS in England. Scotland has its own web-based multiprofessional preceptorship programme called Flying Start NHS (**www.flyingstart. scot.nhs.uk/**) and the Welsh and Northern Ireland Assemblies both support the use of preceptorship for new registrants during their first year although they have not adopted a specific framework as yet.

The Framework provides:

- a definition of preceptorship;
- the key elements of good preceptorship;
- suggested benefits of preceptorship;
- standards for preceptorship;
- guidance on developing preceptorship programmes;
- a suggested set of outcome measures;
- a set of pledges for the preceptee, preceptor, employer and strategic health authority.

The suggested content for preceptorship programmes described in the Framework by the Department of Health (2010a) forms the basis for this book:

- confidence in applying evidence-based practice;
- develop confidence and self-awareness;
- implement the codes of professional values;
- increase knowledge and clinical skills;
- integrate prior learning into practice;
- understand policies and procedures;
- reflection and receiving feedback;
- develop an outcome based approach to continuing professional development;
- advocacy;
- interpersonal skills;
- manage risk and not being risk averse;
- equality and diversity;
- negotiation and conflict resolution;
- leadership and management development;
- team-working;
- decision-making.

Flying Start NHS

Flying Start NHS was first developed in Scotland in 2006 as a national development programme for nurses, midwives and allied health professionals to help them manage the transition from student to newly qualified practitioner and develop their learning and confidence (Roxburgh et al., 2010). The Department of Health has worked with NHS Scotland to develop a web-based programme for England (**www.flyingstartengland.nhs.uk**) with ten units of study that allow practitioners to map their progress against the Knowledge and Skills Framework (KSF) and so work towards their developmental review for their NHS KSF foundation gateway at the end of their first year as a registered practitioner.

Each unit of study has a series of activities which you can choose from, depending on your learning needs and learning style and which you can build into a portfolio for use at your KSF six- and 12-month developmental reviews.

The website also has sections for preceptors and managers as well as forums for preceptees and preceptors to enable them to engage with colleagues to share their experiences and provide support to each other. Some NHS employers may decide to use the website as the basis for their preceptorship programme.

The role of the preceptor

A preceptor is defined as *a registered practitioner who has been given a formal responsibility to support a newly registered practitioner through preceptorship* (Department of Health, 2010a, page 6). Your preceptor should be from the same part of the NMC register as you (e.g. adult nurse or mental health nurse, etc.) and have at least one year's experience in the area in which you will be working. While there is no specific course for preceptors, it is expected that most preceptors will have completed a mentorship course and will probably also have a role as a mentor. This can be a challenge for them as while there are many similarities they are also different roles.

The role of your preceptor is primarily to provide you with the support you need to settle into your role as a registered nurse. There is a general consensus in the literature (Department of Health, 2010a; NMC, 2006) on the key elements of the role, which include:

- acting as a role model;
- acting as a teacher and resource to help you develop the skills and knowledge you require;
- identifying your learning needs with you and agreeing a development plan to meet those needs;
- providing feedback on your performance when you do well;
- providing feedback on your performance where you fall short of the expected level of competence in any areas and agreeing a plan to remedy this.

It is important to recognise that while the role of your preceptor will have similarities with that of the mentors you had when you were a student, it is fundamentally different because you are both registered nurses and you are now an employee and potentially a long-term member of the team.

The role of the preceptee

The NMC (2006) preceptor guidelines set out the responsibilities of the new registrant (and therefore the preceptee) by stating that they must:

- practise in accordance with the NMC Code of Professional Conduct: Standards for Conduct, Performance and Ethics;

- identify and meet with their preceptor as soon as is possible after they have taken up the post;
- identify specific learning needs and develop an action plan for addressing these needs;
- ensure that they understand the standard, competencies or objectives set by your employer that they are required to meet;
- reflect on their practice and experience; and
- seek feedback on their performance from their preceptor and those with whom they work (NMC, 2006, page 2).

All of the above will feel very familiar to you as you will have had to do this whilst a student nurse or student on an overseas nursing programme or return to practice programme.

Activity 1.3: Critical thinking

The differences between being a student and a preceptee

Look at the role and responsibilities of a preceptee, listed above. Consider how your responsibilities differ from those in your previous role as a student.

There is a brief outline answer to this activity at the end of the chapter.

The key difference is around your accountability to the NMC, the public and your employer. We will look at accountability in more detail in Chapters 7 and 12. The organisation you work for may have competencies they wish you to achieve as part of your preceptorship programme and which your preceptor will assess you on. Again this process will be familiar to you but the competencies should not be the only focus. You will also need to identify personal objectives that relate to the development of the skills and knowledge you require in your new area of practice and you will need to consider how they link to the knowledge and skills outline for your post to enable you to pass through the foundation gateway.

Agenda for Change and the Knowledge and Skills Framework

In 2004 a new NHS national pay and grading system was introduced known as Agenda for Change (AfC). The aim was to harmonise pay and terms and conditions for all employees in the NHS (excluding doctors and dentists). AfC includes an appraisal and career development framework known as the NHS Knowledge and Skills Framework (KSF) and was adopted by the majority of NHS organisations.

The KSF is a developmental tool that describes the skills and knowledge that are required for each NHS post. Each post will have a KSF outline which is made up of six core dimensions that are applicable to all posts, and up to seven additional specific dimensions. There are 24 specific dimensions which are grouped under four themes: health and wellbeing; estates and facilities; information and knowledge; and general. The six core dimensions are:

1. communication;
2. personal and people development;

3. health, safety and security;
4. service development;
5. quality;
6. equality and diversity.

Each dimension is divided into four levels with the higher levels setting out greater expectations of the knowledge and skills required for the post. A Band 5 staff nurse post is likely to have a mix of level two and three.

At the end of each year you will receive a developmental review to identify whether you have any development needs. For each pay band there are two incremental developmental reviews or gateway reviews. The first occurs 12 months after you have joined a pay band and is known as the foundation gateway. The timing of the second gateway varies depending on the pay band but occurs near the top. The increments you receive at the two gateways are in recognition of the fact that you are fulfilling the KSF outline for your post. If you are not meeting the outline you cannot receive your increment at that point. However, there should never be any surprises at your gateway review. If there have been any concerns regarding your ability to apply the knowledge and skills set out in the KSF outline they have to be raised at the time in order that they can be addressed.

The Knowledge and Skills Framework and foundation gateway for Band 5

During your first year as a Band 5 nurse, you will have two developmental reviews which will allow for an accelerated progression through the first two points of the pay scales provided you have demonstrated that you are applying the knowledge and skills set out in your KSF outline. Preceptorship is seen as essential to support you through this first year.

The first developmental review is at six months; you can liken it to the mid-point interview when you were a student. The aim is to ensure that you are on the right track to meet the requirements to pass the foundation gateway after 12 months in employment and if so you will receive your first incremental point on the pay scale for a Band 5 post at that six-month point.

You should have received a copy of the KSF outline for your post and before the end of 12 months you will receive a developmental review focusing on this KSF outline which forms your foundation gateway. When you move through this gateway you move up yet another increment on your pay scale (The NHS Staff Council, 2010). The KSF personal development review is explored in more depth in Chapter 17.

Case study: Gina's first month as a preceptee

My first month absolutely whizzed by. I had worked here on my final placement and knew my preceptor Tom as he'd been my sign-off mentor. We had sat down after the first week and discussed my areas of strength and areas I needed to work on and agreed a personal development plan. This was easy to do because Tom knew me and so I felt comfortable in disclosing my fears to him and he knew what I was

continued overleaf...

continued... ••

capable of. We identified that I needed to develop confidence in medicines management, how to delegate care to other members of the team and to develop a number of clinical skills specific to the area. He reminded me that he wouldn't be closely supervising me as when I was a student, which made me feel a bit nervous at first. However, we agreed what my responsibilities were with regards to the areas I needed to develop, which was to make sure I undertook at least three drug rounds per week with a small group of clients, practise for my medicines management test for IV administration and to undertake some reading around the clinical skills I was unsure of. Tom agreed to meet with me every two weeks initially to check on my progress and to spend a little time to reflect with me on my delegation skills. This really gave me the confidence I needed, knowing he was there for me if I needed him.

Chapter summary

Your first year as a newly registered nurse and preceptee is the start of what we hope will be a long and fulfilling career as a nurse. It is also the continuation of a lifetime of learning. Your preceptor will play an important role in helping you with your transition but more important is your realisation that you are now responsible and accountable for your actions and inactions and therefore you must actively seek help when you require support and guidance and not wait for others to tell you what to do.

Activities: brief outline answers

Activity 1.1: Identifying your fears (page 6)

These will be personal to you. However, take a look at the list below, which identifies the fears and worries that Higgens et al. (2010) found newly registered nurses experienced when starting out in their first post:

- feeling terrified, scared to death, a sense of drowning or feeling overwhelmed;
- loss of confidence with regards to skills and knowledge;
- worries around medication management;
- being responsible and accountable;
- delegating care to students and healthcare assistants;
- managing expectations of the team you are joining;
- failing to provide safe care to patients/clients;
- fears of litigation;
- maintaining the standards of care you had been taught in university;
- prioritising care needs and time management;
- decision-making.

You are not alone therefore in your fears and it is important that you discuss your worries with your preceptor.

Activity 1.2: The benefits of preceptorship (page 7)

Your answer will be personal to you and may well include some specific skills and knowledge related to the area in which you are working. The Department of Health's Preceptorship Framework (2010a) suggests that preceptorship develops the following for the preceptee:

- confidence;
- professional socialisation into the working environment;
- increased job satisfaction leading to improved patient/client/service user satisfaction;
- feels valued and respected by their employing organisation;
- feels invested in and enhances future career aspirations;
- feels proud and committed to the organisation's corporate strategy and objectives;
- understanding of the commitment to working within the profession and regulatory body requirements;
- personal responsibility for maintaining up-to-date knowledge.

Activity 1.3: The differences between being a student and a preceptee (page 10)

Your first response may be that there is very little difference from your responsibilities when you were a student. However, there is one very obvious difference in that you are now a registered nurse and so accountable for your actions. You will also notice that there is a greater onus on you to be proactive in identifying your learning needs and to seek help and support.

Further reading

Department of Health (2010a) *Preceptorship Framework for Newly Registered Nurses, Midwives and Allied Health Professionals*, available at **www.dh.gov.uk/prod_consum_dh/groups/dh_digitalassets/@ dh/@en/@abous/documents/digitalasset/dh_114116.pdf**, last accessed 5 July 2010.

Useful websites

www.flyingstart.scot.nhs.uk/
Flying Start NHS (Scotland)

www.flyingstartengland.nhs.uk/
Flying Start England
These websites provide online development programmes for all newly registered nurses in Scotland and England. Throughout this book there will be suggested links to a variety of online activities that complement the content of each chapter.

www.nhsemployers.org
NHS Employers

www.rcn.org.uk
Royal College of Nursing

Chapter 2
Developing confidence and self-awareness

Preceptorship Framework and KSF

This chapter maps to the following elements of the Department of Health Preceptorship Framework and the NHS Knowledge and Skills Framework.

Preceptorship Framework
- Develop confidence and self-awareness
- Increase knowledge and clinical skills
- Integrate prior learning into practice
- Personal and people development
- Quality

NHS Knowledge and Skills Framework
- Communication

Chapter aims

The aim of this chapter is to assist you to identify specific learning and professional development needs that will underpin your preceptorship programme. By the end of this chapter you will be able to:

- undertake a self-assessment in order to identify your learning needs;
- identify your current learning style and use this to implement adult learning strategies;
- utilise strategies to promote self-awareness of your developmental needs.

Introduction: where am I?

In the last chapter we explored the concept of preceptorship and various expectations of you as you progress through your first year as a registered nurse. By now you should have a very clear understanding of the Preceptorship Framework outlined by the Department of Health, and also the role of your preceptor as you undertake your preceptorship programme.

As discussed in the previous chapter, there is no one standardised course or preceptorship programme in the UK. While some organisations may use elements of Flying Start NHS (Scotland) or Flying Start England to facilitate your programme, other organisations may choose to design and facilitate a bespoke preceptorship programme that meets particular local objectives. Either approach is acceptable, as long as the programme satisfies the requirement of the Department of Health *Preceptorship Framework for Newly Registered Nurses, Midwives and Allied Health Professionals*, published in March 2010.

Standards of competence

While there can be considerable flexibility and variation in the preceptorship programme you are undertaking, there is no such flexibility in the competence expected of you as a registered nurse. As we discussed in the previous chapter, the Knowledge and Skills Framework includes explicit requirements for all core competencies and these are not negotiable. Your organisation will have determined the appropriate level of competency expected of you for each core element, and you will be expected to demonstrate this evidence of competence in order to progress through your foundation gateway.

Great expectations

Now that you are a registered nurse it will be expected that you will have no difficulty in demonstrating the appropriate level of competence throughout your preceptorship programme. Your organisation will have invested considerable time and money recruiting you into their organisation, and they will expect a return for their investment. The good news is that you really are wanted. Take pride in the fact that you were employed into your post because your employer believes you will be an asset to their organisation. Your new employer wants the best for you and from you; and they want you to experience a quick and smooth transition from being a student nurse to working with minimal supervision as a registered nurse. Take it as a complement that you have been identified as someone who will be able to take on the challenges of professional development and assume increasing responsibility as you make that transition.

Activity 2.1: Team-working

Identifying skill mix

One of the more confusing aspects of starting any new role is identifying where you fit within the organisation. This activity is to help you identify the current skill mix of nursing staff in your practice area. By completing the activity you should begin to understand your place within the skill mix and develop your self-awareness. You should also begin to identify the people within your immediate practice area who will be able to support you during your preceptorship year.

Use the grid below to write in all the nursing staff within your practice area. You may need the help of your manager to ensure you are accurate, or look at a current staff rota. Identify what Agenda for Change (AfC) band each nurse fits into.

As a newly registered nurse you will obviously be included within the Band 5 numbers. Take some time to reflect on where you fit into this team. Who would you be able to call on for advice and support? Who is likely to be able to answer questions and clarify

continued overleaf...

continued... information? You may even find it useful to ask your manager how many newly qualified Band 5 posts your practice area can support at any one time and if there are other newly registered nurses in your work area.

Colleagues' names	Role and responsibility	Band

There is a brief outline answer to this activity at the end of the chapter.

Expectations of learning

One of the biggest challenges facing newly registered nurses is in taking ownership of your own professional development. While your organisation will usually be facilitating a preceptorship programme for you, a large proportion of that programme will probably involve self-directed learning, perhaps via e-learning materials, workbooks, reflective exercises or self-study activities. You will be given the opportunity to learn independently in certain areas without the need for constant formalised tuition (Timmins, 2008). This is because it will be assumed that you have all the qualities of an adult learner. In fact, you will have needed to provide evidence of these qualities in order to demonstrate the proficiency required for entry to the register. In general, the core principles of an adult learner are as follows:

- the adult learner wants to be self-directed;
- the adult learner accumulates over time a reservoir of experience;
- the adult learner has a readiness to learn;
- the adult learner is aware of their own learning needs;
- the adult learner is motivated to learn (Knowles et al., 1998).

It will be assumed that as a registered nurse you possess all of these qualities and that you will be able to engage with learning activities that rely on pre-existing adult learning skills.

Time to study

If your preceptorship programme is linked to a credit-based academic course of study then you may be allocated some study leave to undertake the programme. It may be that study leave is isolated to the taught elements of your course. However, if it is a locally run programme facilitated 'in house' then any study leave will be entirely at the discretion of your organisation. It is unrealistic to expect that you will be provided with paid study leave for all elements of your preceptorship programme. No doubt there will be opportunities for tutorial sessions and face-to-face discussions; however, you may find that part or the entire self-directed element of your preceptorship programme is your personal responsibility. Your organisation will expect you as an adult learner to be responsible for allocating an appropriate amount of time to develop your knowledge and skills. Of course, as a registered nurse you are professionally obligated to keep your knowledge and skills up to date. This is viewed by the Nursing and Midwifery Council (NMC) as a professional responsibility and there is no fixed requirement for your organisation to provide you with study leave for all professional development activities. The NMC outlines that in terms of your professional development you are required to:

*   keep your knowledge and skills up to date throughout your working life;
*   take part in appropriate learning and practice activities that maintain and develop your competence and performance (NMC, 2008a).

Motivation for learning

Self-directed learning takes considerable motivation. If you are undertaking a preceptorship programme that links to a credit-based academic course then there will be some incentive related to a mark or grade. However, if you are undertaking an 'in house' preceptorship programme then you will be expected to take responsibility for your professional development without the incentive of a grade or award to drive motivation. While there may be some formal assessment events during your preceptorship programme these will not be linked to marks or grades, and in many cases the assessment will be graded on a pass or fail basis. In addition, you will probably be expected to prepare for assessments during your own time, fitted around your normal duty rota, with only limited access to formal feedback. Many newly registered nurses find that the expectation to perform competently within a short period without constant tutorial feedback and reassurance can be one of the most difficult aspects of adjusting to the role (Olson, 2009). You will therefore need considerable motivation and focus to ensure that you do commit sufficient time to your professional development needs.

Case study: Simon discusses motivation during preceptorship

I qualified as a nurse last year and I was fortunate to get my first job straight out of university. I found the preceptorship programme brilliant, but it did take some time to adjust to how different it was to university. I remember sitting a drug calculation test and I really hadn't put much time into studying for it. I didn't do well at all and when they told me I had failed on my first attempt I was really disappointed. At the time I think I was still in student mode and tried to blame my manager on not giving me time to study. My preceptor was more realistic though and just pointed out that if I wanted to pass then I should have put the effort into studying. He explained that it's just not realistic for nurses to have constant time off to study as there would be no one left to care for the clients. It made me realise that I have different obligations now; I'm not supernumerary any more and client care will always have to come before personal study.

Simon learned the hard way about finding motivation. If you were reliant on grades, formal feedback or personal tutor support to generate your motivation as a student nurse you will need to establish alternative ways to maintain motivation throughout your preceptorship programme. You will need to keep in mind that motivation for seeking out and engaging with learning experiences can wane if it is rooted in *extrinsic* motivational forces rather than grounded within *intrinsic* aspects of your personality (Sharples, 2009). Just like Simon in the case study above, it may take some time to accept that your supernumerary status no longer applies. As a registered nurse you will need to accept your own responsibility for learning, and to enact a learning plan you will need to be motivated enough to negotiate your learning needs (Begley and Brady, 2002).

The secret is to develop a new strategy for learning that fits into your current situation. For example, rather than being motivated to achieve a grade of 70%, you could redirect your motivation towards something more practical, like demonstrating that you can lead a team meeting or ward round. In Chapter 4 we will look at the relationship between motivation and learning plans in far more detail.

Developing self-awareness

Your first year as a registered nurse will be a challenging experience. Most newly registered nurses experience a degree of what is commonly referred to as culture shock, where the world of work is quite different to that which they have experienced through student eyes (Godinez et al., 1999). You will need to acknowledge that you are in a process of transition, adapting to a major life change. It is not uncommon to feel quite lost as you move through this transition. While the excitement of gaining your first post as a registered nurse cannot be underestimated, it is also quite normal to feel sad as you will have lost your previous place of security. You will have 'lost' university friends, faculty support and familiarity of routine and may even experience symptoms of grief such as anxiety and depression (Schoessler and Waldo, 2006).

Case study: Claire reflects on being a newly qualified nurse

In my first three months as a registered nurse I put so much pressure on myself trying to be perfect. I just felt I had to know everything. I was trying so hard to fit in and appear confident, but on the inside I was petrified and felt constantly out of my depth. I was barely sleeping, worrying constantly about making a mistake. My manager took me aside and explained that it was alright to ask for help, and that I should communicate if I was unsure or finding particular parts of the job difficult. She also explained that it was OK to tell my patients that I was newly qualified, and they would also be understanding and supportive as I found my feet. I realised that in pretending everything was OK, I was actually stopping people from giving me the help and support I needed. My 'act' that I was confident meant that everyone just assumed I was coping. The breakthrough came when I accepted that I didn't have to pretend to know everything. My attitude just changed overnight, as I found the confidence to ask for help and support when I needed it and stopped treating this as failure.

Try not to place unrealistic expectations on yourself as you move through this transitional period. It is understandable that you will feel a degree of disorientation as you adjust to the demands of being a registered nurse. For a time you may feel as if you are in a state of limbo; the rules of being a student will no longer be applicable to you, yet the rules of the healthcare setting will feel strange and unfamiliar (Schoessler and Waldo, 2006). In the case study above Claire found it difficult to ask for help as she didn't want to seem as if she was still a student asking her mentor for help. However, she did need help and advice in some situations and was putting far too much pressure on herself to be perfect. It is important that you are aware of your own feelings and are willing to acknowledge that at times you will feel overwhelmed and lack confidence in your own ability (Hobbs and Green, 2003). Self-awareness will be essential as you move through your preceptorship year; not only will you gain insight into your development needs but you will be able to share your concerns and anxieties with those who can offer support.

Self-awareness and self-assessment

Self-awareness during your preceptorship year will require regular self-assessment to ensure you are aware of your own development needs. You should already be familiar with self-assessment and using self-assessment tools so you can easily transfer these skills into your preceptorship programme. In essence there are two important areas of self-awareness/self-assessment that you should utilise. Firstly, you will need to be aware of your own learning style. There are many learning style questionnaires available that can help you to understand your own particular style of learning. The Learning Style Questionnaire developed by Honey and Mumford (1992) is one such example that can be used for identifying your learning style (a link can be found in Useful websites at the end of the chapter). The four different learning styles explain not only a preference for a style of learning, but also personality traits that explain preferences for certain experiences over others. It is worth looking at each of the different styles as you may recognise some attributes to be an accurate description of you, both your likes and your dislikes (Sharples, 2009). You will need a clear understanding of your style of learning as different styles suit different situations and you will need to develop the skills to use all four styles in order to take advantage of all the professional development opportunities throughout your preceptorship year.

Concept summary: Honey and Mumford learning styles

Activists

Activists involve themselves fully and without bias in new experiences. They enjoy the here and now and are happy to be dominated by immediate experiences. They are open-minded, not sceptical, and this tends to make them enthusiastic about anything new. Their philosophy is 'I'll try anything once'. They tend to act first and consider the consequences afterwards. Their days are filled with activity. They tackle problems by brainstorming. As soon as the excitement from one activity has died down, they are busy looking for the next. They tend to thrive on the challenge of new experiences but are bored with implementation and longer-term consolidation. They are gregarious people constantly

continued overleaf...

continued...

involving themselves with others but, in doing so, they seek to centre all activities around themselves.

Reflectors

Reflectors like to stand back and ponder experiences and observe them from many different perspectives. They collect data, both first hand and from others, and prefer to think about it thoroughly before coming to any conclusion. The thorough collection and analysis of data about experiences and events is what counts so they tend to postpone reaching definitive conclusions for as long as possible. Their philosophy is to be cautious. They are thoughtful people who like to consider all possible angles and implications before making a move. They prefer to take a back seat in meetings and discussions. They enjoy observing other people in action. They listen to others and get the drift of the discussion before making their own points. They tend to adopt a low profile and tend to have a slightly distant, tolerant, unruffled air about them. When they act it is part of a wide picture which includes the past as well as the present and others' observations as well as their own.

Theorists

Theorists adapt and integrate observations into complex but logically sound theories. They think through problems in a vertical, step-by-step, logical way. They assimilate disparate facts into coherent theories. They tend to be perfectionists who won't rest easy until things are tidy and fit into a rational scheme. They like to analyse and synthesise. They are keen on basic assumptions, principles, theories, models and systems thinking. Their philosophy prizes rationality and logic: 'if it's logical it's good'. Questions they frequently ask are: 'Does it make sense?' 'How does this fit with that?' 'What are the basic assumptions?' They tend to be detached, analytical and dedicated to rational objectivity rather than anything subjective or ambiguous. Their approach to problems is constantly logical. This is their 'mental set' and they rigidly reject anything that doesn't fit with it. They prefer to maximise certainty and feel uncomfortable with subjective judgements, lateral thinking and anything flippant.

Pragmatists

Pragmatists are keen on trying out ideas, theories and techniques to see if they work in practice. They positively search out new ideas and take the first opportunity to experiment with applications. They are the sort of people who return from management courses brimming with new ideas that they want to try out in practice. They want to get on with things and act quickly and confidently on ideas that attract them. They tend to be impatient with ruminating and open-ended discussions. They are essentially practical, down-to-earth people who like making practical decisions and solving problems. They respond to problems and opportunities 'as a challenge'. Their philosophy is 'There is always a better way' and 'If it works it's good'. (Honey and Mumford, 1992, pages 5–6)

Activity 2.2: Critical thinking

Identifying your learning style

After reading through the explanation of the Honey and Mumford learning styles, you will have identified the learning style that is most like yours, and also the style that is least like yours. While it is understandable that you will have a preferred style for learning, one of the skills you constantly develop as a registered nurse is to use all learning styles within your professional practice. The grid below provides an opportunity to match aspects of nursing care with learning styles. Copy this grid and include space in which to match each of the learning styles with some example of nursing care they relate to.

Learning style	Nursing care
Activist	What aspects of nursing care will appeal to an activist?
Reflector	What aspects of nursing care will appeal to a reflector?
Theorist	What aspects of nursing care will appeal to a theorist?
Pragmatist	What aspects of nursing care will appeal to a pragmatist?

There is a brief outline answer to this activity at the end of the chapter.

In addition to understanding your learning style you will need to be confident in using a self-assessment tool to identify your strengths and weaknesses so you can decide on a strategy for your professional development. A SWOT analysis is an effective way of identifying your strengths and weaknesses, and of examining the opportunities and threats you face. Undertaking a SWOT analysis will provide a framework to focus your activities on the areas where you are strongest and also where your greatest challenges and obstacles will lie (Pearce, 2007).

Activity 2.3: Critical thinking

Carrying out a SWOT analysis

Use the grid below to undertake a SWOT analysis of your current activities. There are suggestions in each box on the types of areas you could focus on as you consider your professional development needs. You may find it helpful to refer to your job description and/or KSF outline to develop this activity.

Strengths: What do you do well? Consider this from your point of view and also ask the advice of your preceptor and those you work with.	**Weaknesses: What do you need to improve on?** Consider this from your point of view and also ask the advice of your preceptor and those you work with.

continued overleaf...

continued...

| Opportunities: What current opportunities are available for professional development? Consider support within your organisation and your learning strengths. | Threats: What obstacles confront you? Consider specific obstacles; for example, personal weaknesses or particular learning needs, both knowledge and skills (time constraints? conflicts with colleagues? personal/ home issues?). |

Adapted from Pearce (2007).

There is a brief outline answer to this activity at the end of the chapter.

SWOT analysis and professional development

No doubt you will have particular learning and development needs as you begin your preceptorship programme. However, these will not remain stagnant: you will constantly be changing and developing throughout your first year as a registered nurse. Try to get into the habit of undertaking a fresh SWOT analysis every two to three months, bearing in mind feedback from both colleagues and patients. Not only will you be able to remain focused on your current developmental priorities, you will also be able to track your progress as weaknesses turn into strengths, and threats turn into opportunities.

Chapter summary

Throughout this chapter we have discussed the range of tools that will support your professional development during your preceptorship programme. However, the key to success during your preceptorship year will be your attitude and commitment to your own learning needs. During your programme you will need to frequently participate in self-assessment in order to identify your learning needs. Critically, you will need to implement adult learning strategies in order to make use of the development experiences available to you.

Activities: brief outline answers

Activity 2.1: Identifying skill mix (page 15)

This activity allows you to understand your place within the skill mix and develop your self-awareness of your role within your current practice area. You should also begin to identify the people within your immediate practice who will be able to support you during your preceptorship year. A sample of what this may look like is below:

Colleagues' names	Role and responsibility	Band
Jane Fellows	The ward manager. Has been manager here for six years. Works Mon–Fri, always a morning shift. Has excellent knowledge and skills.	Band 7
Peter Kelly	Charge nurse. Has been a registered nurse for four years, new to this post three months ago. Works full time. Is the education link for students.	Band 6
Marie Connelly	Sister. Has worked on the ward for 14 years. Works part-time two long days a week. Is my preceptor and is willing to answer all questions.	Band 6
Naima Patel	Staff nurse. Has worked on the ward for two years. Always seems very busy. Less approachable to ask questions.	Band 5
Gloria Owusu	Staff nurse. Has worked on the ward for three years. Just back from maternity leave. Works full time. Very friendly but finding it difficult to settle back to work.	Band 5
Glen Thomas	Healthcare assistant. Has worked on the ward for three years. Works part time. Very friendly and very good team member.	Band 3
Valerie Gordon	Healthcare assistant. Has worked on the ward for 12 years. Difficult to approach.	Band 3

While this is just a sample list it should give you an idea of the sort of information you may find useful when completing this activity for yourself.

Activity 2.2: Identifying your learning style (page 21)

This activity allowed you to review nursing care according to the different types of learning styles they may appeal to. Some examples of this are provided in this answer:

Learning style	Nursing care
Activist	• Care of critically ill patients • Bed management issues • Wound care • Diffusing conflict • Emergency situations
Reflector	• Developing and following protocols • Multidisciplinary team meetings • Ward rounds • Record-keeping • Handover
Theorist	• Discharge planning • Drug calculations • Use of risk assessment tools • Care planning

Learning style	Nursing care
Pragmatist	• Airway management • Pre- and post-operative care • Infection control procedures • Medication administration • Referrals to community services

Activity 2.3: Carrying out a SWOT analysis (page 21)

This activity promotes self-awareness through looking at specific aspects of your professional development. An example may look as follows:

Strengths: What do you do well? Communication with patients. I'm confident with this and my preceptor agrees that patients find me easy to understand and I am able to build a rapport easily.	**Weaknesses: What do you need to improve on?** I get very nervous when I have to discuss patient care in meetings. I forget information and need prompting to remember.
Opportunities: What current opportunities are available for professional development? My preceptor has offered to work with me to design a template for these meetings so I learn to systematically hand over the information. This will help me to gain confidence.	**Threats: What obstacles confront you?** I'm worried that people will laugh at me for using the template to remember.

Further reading

Pearce, C (2007) Ten steps to carrying out a SWOT analysis. *Nursing Management*, 14 (2): 25.
This brief article provides a very succinct overview of the SWOT framework and how it can be applied to practice.

Useful websites

The Honey and Mumford learning styles questionnaire is a valuable tool to identify your learning style. The full questionnaire is available at: **www.peterhoney.com**.

To further your self-awareness you may find it beneficial to undertake the *How do I contribute to my team?* activity available on the Flying Start England website. You will find the details of this activity at: **www.flyingstartengland.nhs.uk/teamwork/rolesandcontributions**

To develop your confidence in communicating within a team you may find the 'Communication challenges for individuals' activity on the Flying Start NHS website useful to complete. You will find the details of this activity at: **www.flyingstart.scot.nhs.uk/learning-programmes/communication/interpersonal-skills.aspx#1234**

Chapter 3
Reflection and receiving feedback

Preceptorship Framework and KSF

This chapter maps to the following elements of the Department of Health Preceptorship Framework and the NHS Knowledge and Skills Framework.

Preceptorship Framework

- Reflection and receiving feedback
- Develop confidence and self-awareness
- Increase knowledge and clinical skills
- Integrate prior learning into practice

NHS Knowledge and Skills Framework

- Communication
- Personal and people development
- Quality

Chapter aims

The aim of this chapter is to assist you to explore the use of reflection and feedback to support your professional development. By the end of this chapter you will be able to:

- select the model of reflection that may be most appropriate for you to use in a practice setting;
- develop confidence in seeking and receiving feedback on your performance in practice;
- identify links between self-awareness and reflection in relation to professional development.

Introduction: learning through reflection

As a newly registered nurse the concept of using reflection to learn should be very familiar to you. As a student you will have looked at reflective models and used reflection to learn from your experiences to develop learning goals. You will take these same skills with you throughout your entire nursing career. During your preceptorship programme it will be essential that you employ a reliable reflective model to guide your experience and professional development. As reflection will be rooted in your experiences you will need to make sense of these experiences in order to pinpoint specific learning needs. In fact, the SWOT analysis activity that you undertook in the previous chapter was only possible by reflecting on your experience and current situation.

As you repeat the SWOT analysis activity throughout your preceptorship programme you will continually be reflecting on fresh experiences to develop your understanding and chart your progress.

The value of reflection

Let's take some time to revisit reflection and the value of reflection in nursing. As you will already be aware, reflection is a complex and deliberate process of thinking about and interpreting an experience or experiences in order to learn from them (Boud et al., 1985). Reflection is highly personalised, and no two people's reflection on the same event will be the same. The outcome of reflection is often a changed perspective or learning experience. All reflection requires a trigger to start; however, it will usually be something new or different that initiates reflection. As a newly qualified nurse virtually every day will be new or different to begin with, as even familiar aspects of care will seem markedly different with your new accountability and responsibility. You may reflect almost constantly to begin with, both during and after your shift is officially finished. You will find yourself reflecting on everyday aspects of practice, including situations and events which those around you tend to take for granted.

Case study: Ramona discusses her experiences with reflection

When I was at university I remember that we constantly had reflective practice exercises and, to be honest, at the time I thought they were a bit pointless. Then I started my first job and it dawned on me why so much time had been taken up exploring reflection. I went for weeks reflecting over everything I did. The problem was that it wasn't structured reflection, I just worried and 'stewed over' everything that had happened during the day. Sometimes I'd wake up at night worrying about events that had happened on previous shifts, but it didn't actually get me anywhere. Fortunately during my preceptorship programme we went over reflection again and I was able to see how reflection can be positive, and not only can you learn about yourself, but it can help you to be more objective. I learnt that reflection allowed me to debrief and focus on the future rather than the past.

Reflection is vital in nursing as it is intrinsically linked with competency. This is because competency involves not only taking action in practice but learning from practice through reflection (Boud et al., 1985). Reflection changes practice. It challenges events and habitualised, routinised practice and can prevent nurses from becoming complacent, increasing our level of consciousness about all aspects of care (Elcock, 1997). Reflection also plays a vital role in informing practice. It generates new knowledge and/or research and addresses the theory–practice gap so new knowledge may be generated. Lastly, reflection is essential for personal growth and development. Reflection allows us to learn more about ourselves and the way in which we practise (Elcock, 1997). It also provides a mechanism for self-monitoring of practice. It enables nurses to identify the skills they have and those that need to be developed. Atkins and Murphy (1995) suggest that the real value of reflection is that it provides us with the opportunity to utilise more than empirical knowledge and so solves the unique but often complex problems of practice.

Types of reflection

There are many different types of reflection; however, in the context of nursing, there are two types that tend to occur on a day-to-day basis. Reflection in action occurs during clinical events. You will do this unconsciously as you are thinking about a problem or situation while the event is still taking place (Schon, 1983). For example, you will use reflection during a conversation with a patient/client, perhaps altering your language as you reflect on their understanding of the information you are providing.

The second type of reflection is reflection on action. This type of reflection occurs after an event, and is sometimes structured; for example, debriefing about the day's events with a colleague. Schon (1983) contends that reflection on action is more valuable if it is guided as this can ensure that practice is moved forward. Very often, 'nursing intuition' is attributed to the knowledge that has been gained (perhaps even subconsciously) as a result of reflection on action.

As a newly qualified nurse you will use both reflection in action and reflection on action constantly. All clinical actions will be pondered on, during the actual event and afterwards. In fact, just like the experience of Ramona in the previous case study, you may find it difficult to 'switch off' from your work. Be assured that this reaction is quite normal, and stems from the sudden realisation that as a registered nurse you are solely accountable and responsible for your actions and omissions. All newly registered nurses go through this stage, where the security of student days is no longer a reality. It is very important that you make use of your opportunities for reflection during this time. To do this you will need to select a model of reflection that you are comfortable with, and use this model to structure your reflection where possible. Once again, as an adult learner you will be responsible for your own reflection. Remember that the purpose of a reflective model is to learn from your experience and promote professional development. Without a model to structure your reflection you could just find yourself going round and round in circles, reliving practice experiences but not moving forward.

Models of reflection

You will have been introduced to several different models of reflection as a student nurse, so it is quite likely that you already have a preferred model of reflection. Gibbs' reflective model (Gibbs, 1988) is popular amongst students as it is easy to remember and adaptable to a number of different situations. If you are already comfortable with this model there is no need to change.

It is important to remember that there are many different types of reflective models and ways of reflecting. For example, Johns' (2004) model of reflection uses Carper's (1978) theories about ways of knowing and nursing knowledge as a basis for reflection. The most important aspect of reflection is that you choose a model that suits your needs and use it to facilitate your learning. You may find that as you develop your own professional understanding your preference for a reflective model may also change. Which model you decide upon matters little; the most important thing is that you regularly review key elements of your professional practice using a reflective framework.

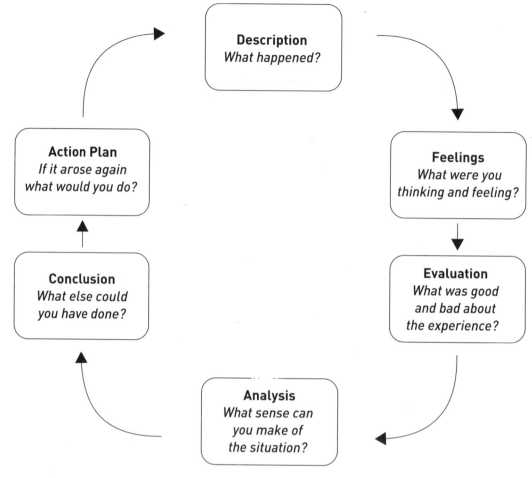

Figure 3.1: Gibbs' reflective model (from Gibbs, 1988)

Case study: Debbie speaks about her use of reflection as a health visitor

Part of my role involves co-ordinating team meetings where we discuss safeguarding of children issues. At the end of each meeting I make sure that we all participate in a structured reflection. This is really useful for new members of the team. Some of the situations that we deal with are very emotionally draining, and we use reflection as a way to debrief as a team but also to ensure that we have an opportunity of reviewing our practice and improving our service. I remember on one occasion during a structured reflection we became aware as a team that we had all felt increased pressure in our roles as a result of a high media profile case. We were able to reflect on how this case had affected us all individually and the fact that our stress levels were very high. It made such a difference for us to acknowledge that we were all feeling the same. We put in an action plan to ensure that we would formally discuss future high profile cases together as part of our weekly meeting. The difference in the room was immediate; it was as if the pressure had been turned off, simply by using reflection to look at our practice and agree a proactive solution.

Activity 3.1: Reflection

A framework for reflection

The following activity provides a formal framework for undertaking a structured reflection. Use this framework now to reflect on an incident or experience that has made an impact on your practice. At the end of this chapter there is an example of how this reflective framework may be used.

1. Describe the incident, issue or situation.
    *   What happened or did not happen?
    *   Who was involved?
    *   How did you behave? How did others behave?
    *   How did you and others feel about the situation?

2. Making sense of the experience.
    *   What factors influenced your actions and the actions of others (consider your own level of knowledge and skills and your feelings about the situation and the people involved as well as other factors such as time, priorities and organisational politics)?

3. What have I learnt?
    *   About me – knowledge or skills deficit or a particular expertise you hold.
    *   About others.
    *   About the organisation.
    *   How will this new knowledge influence me in the future?

4. Formulate an action plan.
    *   What actions will you take to resolve the situation described?
    *   What might the consequences of those actions be? (from Elcock, 2008).

There is a brief outline answer to this activity at the end of the chapter.

Formal reflection

It may be that part of your preceptorship programme provides an opportunity to meet with other newly qualified nurses and reflect on your experiences together. Use these opportunities to share experiences and develop your professional practice. Very often, formal reflective situations like this can reinforce the realisation that you are not as isolated as you may feel, and that others are also finding challenges in adjusting to the demands of being a registered nurse. These discussions can be a great way to debrief in a supportive environment and learn from others who are facing the same challenges as you. These types of discussion are often facilitated by someone within the organisation with the responsibility of managing the preceptorship programme. You may even find that a reflective model is used to structure these discussions.

Keeping a reflective journal

Another way to reflect is by keeping a reflective journal (Elcock, 2008). This does not have to be time-consuming, and like any other skill, it will become easier and quicker to complete the more you do it. Once again you can use a reflective model or framework to structure your thoughts. This can be particularly valuable if you find it difficult to know where to begin. You will probably find that as you become more experienced with reflecting during your preceptorship year, you become less dependent on a formal model.

Tips for keeping a reflective journal

1. Use a loose leaf folder or specific book to record your entries in.
2. If new to journaling use a model/framework to structure your entries.
3. Pre-print/copy several copies of the model or framework with suitable gaps to fill in and put in your folder ready for use.
4. Have it at hand so you don't need to search for it.
5. Identify a time in your day/week when you have space to complete it.
6. Aim to make a minimum of one entry per week.
7. If something happens at work that you think is important or affects you strongly, write down the key points and put the list in your journal until you have time to write it out in full.
8. Try to balance any 'negative' entries with positive ones (from Elcock, 2008).

As an adult learner it will be expected that the majority of your 'reflective learning' will be initiated by you. Keep in mind that while it may not always be possible to arrange formal reflection due to the busyness of practice areas, in most situations it will be possible to undertake informal reflection (Sharples, 2009). You may choose to do this in isolation via a journal, or perhaps reflect in action or on action with your preceptor. Don't be afraid to initiate reflection, even if it's just sharing your feelings over a cup of tea.

Learning through feedback

While reflection is a vital aspect of learning and professional development during your preceptorship programme, it is only really valuable if supported with feedback. While you adjust to being a registered nurse you may be increasingly reliant on your preceptor to guide and encourage you through this experience. The way they will do this is through feedback on your performance.

Once again you should be quite used to receiving feedback, as this would have been a frequent event as a student nurse. During your preceptorship programme, however, you will be receiving feedback on your performance as a registered nurse, and this time the feedback will be linked to the core competencies expected of you to move through your foundation gateway. The bar will therefore be raised quite significantly.

Who will give me feedback?

During your first year as a registered nurse you will receive feedback on your performance from a wide range of sources. Some feedback will be structured and come from designated people charged with this role. For example, your preceptor and preceptor programme facilitators will have the responsibility of providing you with formal feedback during your programme. You can expect that some of this feedback will be documented, perhaps in a professional development portfolio.

However, you will also receive spontaneous, unsolicited feedback from a wide range of sources. Managers, colleagues, clients/patients, relatives, etc., will provide continual feedback. Some feedback you receive will be positive and can be very motivating. However, you can also expect that some feedback will indicate that improvement is needed. You should expect and prepare yourself for this. In fact, without feedback on your weaknesses it will be very difficult to improve the level of your performance. The better you are at understanding and accepting constructive feedback about your performance, the quicker you will be able to make the necessary adjustments to improve. Keep in mind that while reflection is a valuable way to gain insight into your strengths and weaknesses, you are not always the best judge of yourself (Sharples, 2009). In fact, one of the biggest advantages of feedback is that it allows you to gain insight into yourself and learn about yourself.

Research summary: the Johari window

The Johari window is a valuable model that can be used to explore aspects of ourselves and promote self-awareness. It consists of four quadrants:

- open – what we know about ourselves that is also known to others;
- blind – things that others know that we do not;
- hidden – things we know about ourselves but do not reveal to others;
- unknown – unknown to ourselves and others.

The premise of the Johari window is that as we learn more about ourselves the size of the quadrants alter. The more we reveal about ourselves, or the more we become aware of our blind area, the more our unknown area will shrink. While this process develops self-awareness it also means that we must be prepared to receive feedback from others (adapted from Luft (1969) *and* Jack and Smith (2007)).

Activity 3.2: Clinical decision-making

Johari window

In Chapter 2 you were introduced to a SWOT analysis as a way of self-assessing. This activity requires you to use feedback as a means of reflecting and developing your self-awareness. In order to do this you will need to undertake the Johari window activity with your preceptor. You might like to choose a particular area of professional development that you need to focus on during your preceptor programme. We have chosen an example to get you started.

continued overleaf...

continued...

Clinical decision-making

Box 1: In terms of my clinical decision-making, what do I and my preceptor agree on? What I do well and where I need to improve?

Box 2: Has my preceptor noticed any particular strengths or weaknesses in relation to my clinical decision-making that I haven't recognised in myself?

Box 3: Are there any learning needs or difficulties I'm having that my preceptor doesn't know about in relation to my clinical decision-making?

Box 4: Based on the information we've just shared with each other, what do I need to do to improve my clinical decision making?

1. Open Known by self/known by others	**2. Blind** Unknown by self/known by others
3. Hidden Known by self/unknown by others	**4. Unknown** Unknown by self/unknown by others

Adapted from Dennison and Kirk (1990, page 29).

There is a brief outline answer to this activity at the end of the chapter.

Using feedback for professional development

There is a significant link between reflection, feedback and your professional development. As feedback on clinical performance can be a spontaneous part of the working relationship (Eraut, 2006) it will naturally open the door to reflection on practice. Pugh (1992) argues that self-reflection of your performance cannot be underestimated, as it will provide valuable insight into perceptions of your ability. For this reason you should take every opportunity to reflect during feedback situations. Activity 3.2 provides just one example of how this may be facilitated. Your self-reflection should also provide opportunities for a clear discussion on strengths and weaknesses with your preceptor, and help you to regulate your professional development in a realistic way (Glover, 2000). In the next chapter we will begin to look at how self-assessment, reflection and feedback can be utilised to develop learning plans.

Chapter summary

If you have not already done so, invest some time into selecting the model of reflection that you feel comfortable with and are able to adapt to the practice setting. Take every opportunity to reflect on your performance and develop confidence in

continued opposite...

• • *continued...* •

seeking and receiving feedback on your performance in practice. You will be able to use this knowledge to develop your own learning plans to support your professional development.

Activities: brief outline answers

Activity 3.1: A framework for reflection (page 29)

The following outline answer provides an example of how structured reflection may be used within this framework.

1. Describe the incident, issue or situation.
   - What happened or is not happening? (did not happen?)
     I take a very long time to complete a drug round on my ward and I need to improve on this.

   - Who was involved?
     I do the drug round but I also hold other nurses up from their work and patients don't always receive their medications on time.

   - How did you behave? How did others behave?
     I find that the harder I try to be fast the worse it gets. I cried the other day just because I feel under so much pressure.

   - How did you and others feel about the situation?
     I find it really embarrassing that it takes me so long. Some of the registered nurses on my ward are obviously frustrated.

2. Making sense of the experience.
   - What factors influenced your actions and the actions of others (consider your own level of knowledge and skills and your feelings about the situation and the people involved as well as other factors such as time, priorities and organisational politics)?
     I'm trying to prove to everyone that I'm competent but I'm also worried about making a drug error so I check everything over and over again. This slows me down. The other nurses are confident so they are really fast. I also realise that my lack of confidence means that patients don't always get their medications on time and this is really a problem.

3. What have I learnt?
   - About me – knowledge or skills deficit or a particular expertise you hold.
     I want to be perfect but I'm not as confident with medications as I should be.

   - About others.
     I'm part of a team and if I don't improve my confidence then the team and patients are affected.

   - About the organisation.
     The nurses on my ward are willing to help and have offered lots of advice on how to get faster.

   - How will this new knowledge influence me in the future?
     To accept the advice and support I'm offered.

4. Formulate an action plan.
   - What actions will you take to resolve the situation described?
     Speak with my preceptor and try out some strategies for improving speed on drug rounds without affecting accuracy. My ward manager has also offered to help so I need to accept their help rather than try to cope by myself.

   - What might the consequences of those actions be?
     I will improve my confidence in medication rounds by listening and acting on advice. I will be seen as an asset to the team rather than a drain on the team.

Activity 3.2: Johari window (page 31)

An example Johari window based on clinical decision-making is provided below.

Box 1: In terms of my clinical decision-making, what do I and my preceptor agree on in terms of what I do well and where I need to improve?

Box 2: Has my preceptor picked up any particular strengths or weaknesses in relation to my clinical decision-making that I haven't recognised in myself?

Box 3: Are there any learning needs or difficulties I'm having that my preceptor doesn't know about in relation to my clinical decision-making?

Box 4: Based on the information we've just shared with each other, what do I need to do to improve my clinical decision-making?

1. Open

Known by self/known by others
My preceptor and I agree that I lack some confidence when referring clients to the substance misuse service.

2. Blind

Unknown by self/known by others
My preceptor has noticed that I don't experience this lack of confidence when it comes to making day-to-day clinical decisions; however, I need a lot of support in making referrals.

3. Hidden

Known by self/unknown by others
I have dyslexia and this slows me down when documenting notes. I've not told my preceptor about this disability as I'm worried about being stigmatised.

4. Unknown

Unknown by self/unknown by others
If I disclose my dyslexia to my preceptor I will be able to discuss the support I need in documenting client referrals.

Further reading

Johns, C (2004) *Becoming a Reflective Practitioner*, 3rd edn. Oxford: Wiley-Blackwell.

Schon, D (1983) *The Reflective Practitioner: How Professionals Think in Action*. USA: Basic Books.

Useful websites

www.mindtools.com/CommSkill/JohariWindow.htm
This website provides a common-sense, easy approach to understanding the Johari window.

www.becomecoaching.com/documents/GivingEffectiveFeedback.pdf
This easy-to-read PDF summarises the key attributes of constructive feedback and offers practical advice on how to deliver and learn through feedback.

If you are finding it difficult to find time to reflect you may find it beneficial to undertake the practice-based activity available on the Flying Start NHS website. You will find the details of this activity at: **www.flyingstart.scot.nhs.uk/learning-programmes/reflective-practice/reflection.aspx**

If you would like some more practical advice for incorporating reflection into your practice you may like to review 'Top tips for reflecting', available on the Flying Start England website. You will find these tips at: **www.flyingstartengland.nhs.uk/reflective-practice/toptipsforreflecting**

Chapter 4
Integrating prior learning into practice

Preceptorship Framework and KSF

This chapter maps to the following elements of the Department of Health Preceptorship Framework and the NHS Knowledge and Skills Framework.

Preceptorship Framework
- Integrate prior learning into practice
- Develop confidence and self-awareness
- Increase knowledge and clinical skills
- Decision-making

NHS Knowledge and Skills Framework
- Communication
- Personal and people development
- Service improvement
- Quality

Chapter aims

The aim of this chapter is to assist you to identify specific learning and professional development needs based on the outcome of reflection and feedback. By the end of this chapter you will be able to:

- clarify specific learning needs;
- develop learning plans that support your professional development needs;
- identify opportunities for utilising experiential learning within your practice area.

Introduction: planning for success

Achieving the core competencies expected of you during your preceptorship programme will take consistent effort and commitment. The most important factor is that you are honest with yourself regarding your development needs. You will also need to commit time and energy into developing areas that you find challenging. From the very beginning of your preceptorship programme you will need a personal development plan that allows you to focus your efforts on developing all the competencies that will facilitate your transition from academic studies to clinical practice. In

Chapters 2 and 3 we discussed self-awareness, reflection and feedback as methods of identifying areas for professional development. The focus of this chapter will be on using this knowledge to develop learning plans, and identify opportunities for professional development.

What do I need to learn?

Many newly registered nurses make the common error of focusing all their efforts during preceptorship on developing technical competence, and paying less attention to skills in clinical judgement, critical thinking, teamwork, cost awareness, accountability for clinical outcomes and quality of care (Olson, 2009). While it is understandable to want to prove competence in terms of concrete elements and actions, it is important to remember that competence as a registered nurse encapsulates far more than just technical skills. It will be assumed that you have already attained the required core skills in order to justify your fitness to practice. Preceptorship is your opportunity to integrate prior learning into practice and identify areas of weakness that require development. This transition period is your time to learn to manage and control relevant aspects of your practice (Roxburgh et al., 2010). You will therefore be expected to focus on developing independence in your practice via evidence of accountability and responsibility.

Research summary: expected competence of a registered nurse

The competence expected of a newly qualified registered nurse in the UK is determined by the NMC. In 2010 the NMC reviewed the previous *Standards of Proficiency for Pre-registration Nursing Education* (NMC, 2004) and published the *Standards for Pre-registration Nursing Education* (NMC, 2010a). Together with *The Code: Standards of Conduct, Performance and Ethics for Nurses and Midwives* (NMC, 2008a) and *Guidance on Professional Conduct for Nursing and Midwifery Students* (NMC, 2009a), these standards outline the competence required of new nurses completing pre-registration nursing programmes, who are at the point of registration. The NMC makes it very clear that competence is a requirement for entry to the NMC register (NMC, 2010a). The purpose of a preceptorship programme therefore is to provide a platform to integrate pre-existing competence into practice; it is not for the purpose of developing competence that should already exist (Department of Health, 2010a). The NMC does not expect that you will have extensive clinical experience, specialist expertise or have highly developed supervision and leadership skills at the point of registration (NMC, 2010a).

Case study: Carl's experience as a preceptor

A newly registered nurse started in our endoscopy unit about six weeks ago, and I'm so worried about her. She was a very competent student but she has had such a difficult time making the transition to staff nurse. At first we just thought she was really shy, but after a few weeks we realised that her reluctance to get involved wasn't shyness at all. She knows her stuff, there's no question about that, her real problem is that she finds it really difficult to initiate care unless someone gives her permission. It's as if she is still waiting

continued overleaf...

continued...

for her mentor to tell her what to do, or to suggest a way to do it. She is just finding it so difficult to identify what her role is. We have no concerns about her skills or knowledge and she knows that, but she can't seem to make the move to being autonomous. Of course, the longer it goes on the more confidence she loses and you can just see her stress levels rise. We're having a meeting tomorrow to write a specific action plan – I know she can do it, I just want her to realise that.

Being in control

In Chapters 2 and 3 we discussed self-awareness and reflection/feedback at length. One of the many benefits of being self-aware is the degree of control it affords you in relation to your professional development. There is good evidence to support that being unable to exert control over your work will mean that you are more likely to experience work stress, which in turn will impair learning (Taris and Feij, 2004). As a newly registered nurse it is normal to experience a degree of stress; however, if this stress becomes disproportionate you may find psychological barriers to learning, and thus limit your ability to reduce your stress. In the case study above, Carl's preceptee is obviously feeling out of control within her new role, and the stress this causes is actually impeding her from progressing. The key here is to maintain personal control over your learning needs and thereby establish a positive outlet for your stress. You will not be able to do this unless you embrace self-awareness, reflection and feedback as vital tools for your professional development.

Identifying learning needs

By now you should have begun to recognise some clear areas for your professional development that you would like to focus on. To ensure you are focusing on the right areas you should use appropriate tools that we have discussed previously. Ideally you will have a variety of resources such as:

- a reflective journal;
- a variety of SWOT analyses;
- feedback via discussions with your preceptor, perhaps structured through a Johari window.

This information will be vital in order to begin forming learning plans.

Activity 4.1: Critical thinking

Identifying learning needs

The purpose of this activity is to enable you to clarify the specific areas of professional development that you may need to focus on. In order to ensure your learning needs can be clearly identified, it is helpful to categorise them into clear themes. For the purpose of this activity we have chosen to use the Department of Health *Preceptorship Framework for Newly Registered Nurses, Midwives and Allied Health Professionals*, published in March 2010. Next to each theme there is an opportunity to identify specific development needs. Don't

continued opposite...

continued...

feel obligated to identify specific needs in every category; you may only be aware of needs within a selection of categories. Alternatively you could refer to your KSF outline if you have one. As you move through your preceptorship programme you will be developing your self-awareness and insight into your learning needs will follow.

Preceptorship Framework	My development need
Develop confidence and self-awareness	
Reflection and receiving feedback	
Integrate prior learning into practice	
Increase knowledge and clinical skills	
Confidence in applying evidence-based practice	
Understand policies and procedures	
Team-working	
Interpersonal skills	
Advocacy	
Negotiation and conflict resolution	
Implement the Code and professional values	
Manage risk and not being risk averse	
Equality and diversity	
Decision-making	
Leadership and management development	
Develop an outcome-based approach to continuing professional development	

There is a brief outline answer to this activity at the end of the chapter.

Reviewing development needs

At the beginning of each chapter we demonstrate how each theme within the preceptorship framework maps with the six core dimensions of the Knowledge and Skills Framework. By regularly identifying your learning needs in relation to the preceptorship framework, you will also be able to correlate your learning needs within the context of the Knowledge and Skills Framework. As you progress through your preceptorship programme you will constantly be reviewing and revising your development needs. Rather than remaining static, your specific learning needs will fluctuate with time and experience. As Duchscher (2001) explains, your focus during your first six months as a new registrant will be on clinical skills, adjusting to reality and coping. It may be the second six months of your first year that you will become better able to acknowledge higher-order processes such as critical thinking. It is for this reason that you should try to get into the habit of reviewing your learning needs every month to ensure that you are maintaining control over them.

Developing an action plan

In completing Activity 4.1 you should have identified a specific learning need and linked this to a theme within the preceptorship framework. Now it's time to act upon that learning need. In order to do this you will need to develop an action plan or learning contract. This should be very familiar to you, as no doubt action planning/developing a learning contract formed a significant part of your learning as a student. Unfortunately some students view action planning and/or learning contracts as a negative, rather than a positive, aspect of personal development. If you have avoided action plans in the past for this reason, then your preceptorship programme is the time to alter that perspective. Far from being negative, an action plan/learning contract reinforces your control over your learning experience. It provides you with the opportunity for informed choice, time to take your learning seriously and encourages a personal role in your development (Light et al., 2009). The key benefits of action planning include:

- the opportunity to identify specific goals;
- setting goals that are SMART;
- clarifying what is required to achieve goals;
- identifying appropriate resources and strategies that you will need/use;
- an opportunity to gain commitment and support for your learning needs from your preceptor and employer.

Scenario: action planning is positive

Sharon is a registered nurse working in a neurological rehabilitation day care unit. She notices that several of the clients are more irritated than usual on Wednesday mornings, and less likely to concentrate on group activities with the occupational therapist. After noticing this pattern on several Wednesdays, Sharon observes that some clients become more irritable when stock deliveries are taking place. She concludes that unfamiliar faces walking through the group room cause some clients to become distressed and therefore more irritable. Sharon acts on this by notifying all delivery drivers to enter the unit via the side entrance, and to

continued opposite...

continued...

not enter the group room unless escorted by a member of staff that the clients know. This simple change in procedure results in an immediate improvement in concentration among previously distressed clients.

Setting a goal

Sharon was able to use an action plan not only to solve a current problem, but also to reduce the likelihood of future problems. By developing a clear plan of action Sharon was able to take control of the situation, rather than let events control her. The first step in developing an action plan is to establish a clear goal that you would like to achieve. Sometimes this is referred to as a learning objective or learning outcome. These will have formed the basis of your practice assessment as a student. The difference is that as a student learning outcomes were usually prescribed and, as Light et al. (2009) highlight, offered very little space for the development of your own learning. The difference now is that the learning goals you set yourself will be clear statements of what *you* want to achieve. Your learning goals will also be based on what your employer requires you to achieve in order to work successfully as part of the team. In the scenario above Sharon identified a problem and then formulated her own goal of what she wanted to achieve, this being to change the routine of delivery drivers. She designed her own action plan to deal with the situation and made future plans to ensure the problem did not recur. With a clear goal you should not only have a clear direction for learning but also benefit from specific parameters to measure your progress.

Being SMART

For a goal or learning outcome to be effective in the context of your preceptorship programme, it needs to be SMART:

- Specific: accurately state what you want to achieve in terms of your professional development. This may include a specific aspect of knowledge, skills, attitude or values. It could be something that you specifically want to achieve, or specifically wish to avoid.
- Measurable: the goal you wish to achieve must be observable and be linked to an identified aspect of behaviour. For this reason your goal should incorporate action verbs such as plan, select, utilise, apply and demonstrate.
- Achievable: your goals must be within range of your abilities for your current stage of professional development and achievable within your workplace.
- Relevant: relate to the weaknesses highlighted either through formal assessments, feedback, a reflective journal or SWOT analysis.
- Time bound: any goal you set yourself must have clear target dates set for achievement.

Activity 4.2: Critical thinking

Designing a SMART goal

This activity builds on from Activity 4.1 and allows you to identify a SMART goal based on a specific learning need you may have. Try to choose a very straightforward learning

continued overleaf...

continued...

need to begin with so you can master the skill of goal setting very easily. Use the grid below to plan a SMART goal.

Specific	What specific area do you want to focus on?
Measurable	How will you know it has been achieved?
Achievable	Is this something expected of you by this stage of your preceptorship year?
Relevant	What evidence have you got that this needs to be developed?
Time bound	When do you want to achieve your goal by?

There is a brief outline answer to this activity at the end of the chapter.

Accessing resources

Once you have clear goals the actual process of designing an action plan to meet your development needs becomes far more straightforward. An action plan generally has two aspects. The first requires you to identify the resources you need. However, you should not expect that the resources or tools you need to achieve your goal will be automatically given to you. As an adult learner it will be expected that you are able to self-direct your learning and are not reliant on others for constant direction or motivation. You will have spent your time at university learning the skills of a lifelong learner and it will be expected that you possess critical-thinking and problem-solving skills (Brookfield, 1994; Sutherland and Crowther, 2006). In addition, it will be assumed that where there are elements of structured learning you will be able to transfer what you have learned during the structured activity into problem-solving, self-regulation or development of expertise (Zimmerman and Martinez-Pons, 1988).

The resources you need therefore will be largely determined by you; however, this is not to say that you are alone. Remember that you will have access to a range of resources to help you meet your goals. A sample of these may include:

- your preceptor;
- other members of the multidisciplinary team;
- other newly registered nurses;
- formal tutorial events on the preceptorship programme within your organisation;
- informal teaching sessions in your practice area;
- internet/intranet resources (ideal for policy and procedure documents);
- online learning tools (Flying Start NHS/Flying Start England);
- journals and books (like the one you are reading now).

Once you are aware of the resources available, you can begin to plan how to achieve your goals. This is the action part of the plan.

Learning through experience

Previously in this chapter we have identified how to develop a SMART learning goal and the resources that may be called upon in order to achieve the goal. While you may be clear on *what* you want to learn, the second part of an action plan relates to *how* you are going to learn. The most practical, relevant and functional way to do this is by linking your action plan directly into your work experiences. This process is broadly referred to as experiential learning, and refers to a process where there is as an active and interactive process between the learner and the environment (Dewey, 1938).

Experiential learning

The main benefit of an experiential learning cycle is that it allows a learner to engage with a purposeful and realistic way to learn in, from and during the experiences that formulate your daily work. Experiential learning also encourages control over the learning experience, so you can truly feel that you are self-regulating your professional development. Kolb's (1984) process of experiential learning is one of the more popular models as it correlates easily with learning in a nursing context. Kolb's model of experiential learning involves a four-stage cycle that contains four different learning modes (Kolb, 1984). Figure 4.1 shows each stage of the cycle clearly. At each stage of the experiential cycle (concrete experience, reflective observation, abstract conceptualisation and active experimentation) (Kolb, 1984) there is an opportunity to engage with a specific aspect of professional development.

These are as follows:

- concrete experience – an immediate experience that forms the basis of observation and feedback;
- reflective observation – critical reflection;
- abstract conceptualisation – abstract concepts and implications of action;
- active experimentation – goal directed action and evaluation of the consequences (adapted from Light et al., 2009).

Kolb's experiential learning cycle has been criticised for not fully capturing the complexity of the learning process (Jarvis et al., 1998). However, it still provides a solid foundation for active learning and developing new and meaningful experience (Light et al., 2009). Each stage of the cycle flows into the next, promoting a continuum of learning. In the next chapter we will be exploring the experiential cycle in far more detail, with useful links drawn to show how using an experiential cycle promotes acquisition of knowledge and skills. Kolb's learning cycle is explored more fully in Chapter 5.

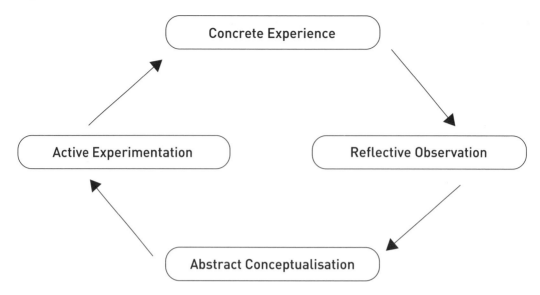

Figure 4.1: Kolb's experiential learning cycle (adapted from Kolb 1984, page 42)

Chapter summary

Throughout this chapter we have discussed the links between self-awareness, reflection/feedback and your current development needs. We established that you commenced your preceptorship programme with your prior learning experience being that of a student. As you progress through your programme you will be integrating not only previous learning, but all your current development as a newly qualified nurse. The aim of this chapter has been to gain an understanding of your current learning needs and to develop learning plans that will support your professional development needs throughout your nursing career. A confident understanding of experiential learning will provide the tools to facilitate this process.

Activities: brief outline answers

Activity 4.1: Identifying learning needs (page 38)

The purpose of this activity was to enable you to clarify the specific areas of professional development that you may need to focus on. An example of one such area is provided below.

Preceptorship Framework	My development need
Understand policies and procedures	The area where I work requires specific infection control practices that I haven't had experience with. I have tried reading the policies but I find them confusing and I keep making mistakes.

Activity 4.2: Designing a SMART goal (page 41)

The focus of this activity was to identify a SMART goal based on a specific learning need you may have. The example provided is based on the learning need identified in the outline answer for Activity 4.1.

Specific	What specific do you want to focus on? *I would like to be able to explain and implement competently the reverse barrier nursing policy for ward G6.*
Measurable	How will you know it has been achieved? *I will know I have achieved this when I can look after any patient requiring reverse barrier nursing without having to ask what I should do or rely on feedback from colleagues.*
Achievable	Is this something expected of you by this stage of your preceptorship year? *All registered nurses on my ward are expected to know this information and my manager has highlighted this as a development need.*
Relevant	What evidence have you got that this needs to be developed? *I made two errors last week in not following the policy and if I don't improve on this then I may cause harm to a patient.*
Time bound	When do you want to achieve your goal? *I would like to achieve this goal in the next week.*

Further reading

Kolb, D (1984) *Experiential Learning: Experience as the Source of Learning and Development.* Englewood Cliffs, New Jersey: Prentice Hall.
This book provides a thorough rationale and explanation of experiential learning for those who wish to explore the origins of Kolb's experiential learning cycle.

Nursing and Midwifery Council (2010) *Standards for Pre-registration Nursing Education.* Available from: **www.nmc-uk.org.**
This latest standard document from the NMC provides an overview of the competencies and essential skills required to enter the professional register from 2012 onwards.

Useful websites

www.positive-thinking-principles.com/action-plan-template.html
This website offers free action plan templates and also valuable examples for using the SMART tool to set personal goals.

If you would like to further assess your development needs you may like to undertake the 'Building confidence' activity on the Flying Start England website. This can be accessed at: **www.flyingstart england.nhs.uk/reflective-practice/confidencebuilding**

You could also use the 'Your NHS KSF post outline' activity on the Flying Start NHS website if you would like to use your PDP to prioritise your learning needs. You will find this activity at: **www. flyingstart.scot.nhs.uk/learning-programmes/cpd/lifelong-learning.aspx**

Chapter 5
Increasing knowledge and clinical skills

Preceptorship Framework and KSF

This chapter maps to the following elements of the Department of Health Preceptorship Framework and the NHS Knowledge and Skills Framework.

Preceptorship Framework
- Increase knowledge and clinical skills
- Integrate prior learning into practice
- Develop confidence and self-awareness
- Team-working

NHS Knowledge and Skills Framework
- Communication
- Personal and people development
- Service improvement
- Quality

Chapter aims

The aim of this chapter is to assist you to recognise the value of professional development opportunities in relation to formal and informal assessment and staff-development events. By the end of this chapter you will be able to:

- prepare for competency testing;
- learn how to use an experiential model to achieve your development goals;
- gain insight into the purpose of peer review/clinical supervision to increase knowledge and skills.

Introduction: promoting knowledge and skills

In the previous chapter we explored the need to identify learning needs in terms of realistic goals and development of action plans. We looked at the rationale behind using an experiential model as a way of achieving desired goals. The purpose of this chapter is to explore the specific ways that experiential learning may be implemented in terms of increasing your knowledge and skills. In order to do this you will need to have a very clear view of the specific areas of knowledge and skills you wish to develop. The previous chapter should have given you insight into how to identify your specific learning needs, set appropriate goals and identify the resources available to you. With this information we can now look specifically at increasing knowledge and skills.

Assessment as a registered nurse

Take some time to think about your recent experience of assessment. During your pre-registration education you will have experienced constant assessment in one form or another. You will have been assessed both formatively and summatively, and assessment will have been undertaken equally in theory and practice. You could quite rightly assume that you are somewhat expert when it comes to assessment. After all, the fact that you are a registered nurse confirms that you have been successful in a multitude of assessments. It may come as quite a shock therefore to find that assessment of your knowledge and skills will be undertaken throughout your preceptorship programme and become an ongoing feature of your nursing career. We will be looking at assessment in far more detail throughout this chapter; however, our starting point will be to ascertain why further assessment is necessary.

Why am I being assessed?

There are two significant factors that need to be addressed in relation to assessment during your preceptorship programme. The first is related to the fact that there are so many different aspects of knowledge and skill required of a registered nurse. As a student nurse it was just not possible to assess you on all variations prior to qualification. For this reason a small sample of competencies will have been assessed as proxies for all (Roberts, 2009). A list of so-called 'sample competencies' may include cardiac resuscitation, personal hygiene, aseptic dressing, hand hygiene and drug administration (Roberts, 2009).

The fact that you have passed these competencies does not automatically imply that you are competent to carry out all aspects of your current role. Let's take medicines management as an example. During your pre-registration programme you will have been required to demonstrate competency in relation to drug calculations. This was probably assessed via simulation and also in practice by mentors. However, because of time limitations your practice experience will have been limited to a sample of practice areas and a sample of practice situations. The fact that you have passed this assessment simply means that you have met the criteria for predictive validity. In other words it is predicted that you will be able to transfer the principles of drug calculations to demonstrate competence in your current practice area. As a newly qualified nurse you will require a further assessment to ensure that you are able to transfer previous knowledge and skill into the specific requirements of your practice area. Within the nursing literature this is widely discussed in terms of 'fitness for purpose' (O'Connor et al., 2001).

Activity 5.1: Reflection

Reviewing specific knowledge and skills

As a pre-registration student you should have maintained some records of the specific areas of knowledge and skill that you were exposed to during your practice experiences.

continued overleaf...

continued...

Take some time now to reflect on the areas of previous experience that relate directly to your current practice area. Now think of specific skills that are undertaken in your practice area that you may not have experienced as a student. We will return to the results of this activity later in the chapter.

There is a brief outline answer to this activity at the end of the chapter.

The second reason that your knowledge and skills will require assessment during your preceptorship programme is because you will be required to demonstrate a different level of knowledge and skill to the standard expected in order to qualify. The limitations on your practice as a student will have prevented you from undertaking some skills required of a registered nurse (Roberts, 2009). Let's return to our previous example of medicines management. To register as a nurse you will have been required to demonstrate competency in relation to drug calculations. However, your status as a student will have meant that you would never have been able to take full accountability and responsibility for the accuracy of that calculation. You will have always been required to check your calculation with at least one registered nurse. Your new status as a registered nurse will require evidence that you can independently perform safe and accurate drug calculations (depending of course on your local policies related to medicines management).

Case study: Claire reflects on her first drug round

During my preceptorship programme I undertook a drug calculation assessment and my preceptor also assessed me administering medications. I was so focused on getting my competencies signed off that I didn't really think too much about what it would mean. I passed all the tests so of course the next day the time came for the usual drug round and my preceptor basically said I was on my own. I remember thinking, 'come back, come back, I'm not ready', but of course that didn't happen. I just remember standing in front of all my patients with a drug trolley open and it just hit me that I was entirely accountable and responsible. I was literally shaking at the thought of what this meant. Of course I was proud to finally be a real nurse and not need someone looking over my shoulder, but it also meant the weight of responsibility was totally with me.

Assessment of competence

At some point during your preceptorship year you can expect to encounter similar feelings to Claire in the case study above. Being a 'real nurse' is something to be very proud of; however, it is also normal to feel very isolated at times. This often occurs when new stages of competency are encountered and you may find yourself practising independently in skills that have previously always been supervised.

During your preceptorship programme there will be instances where specific aspects of knowledge and skill are assessed. It should be very clear by now that the purpose of preceptorship is far more than assessment – as evidenced by the fact that it only accounts for one chapter within this book. However, it will form a part of your programme so it is important to address assessment as a whole.

Throughout your preceptorship programme you will be assessed formatively and summatively and you can expect the assessment to take place through a variety of means. These may include objective structured clinical examination (OSCE), observation in practice and classroom testing. All of these assessment methods should be very familiar to you. If your preceptorship programme is linked to a credit-based academic course of study, this assessment may contribute to a mark or grade. However, if it is a locally run programme facilitated 'in house' then any assessment you undertake will in most cases be marked on a pass/fail criterion.

What will be assessed?

The types and amounts of assessment required during your preceptorship programme are usually dictated by two factors:

- the local competencies required for your role (linked directly to your job description and based upon the knowledge and skills framework);
- whether your preceptorship programme is linked to a credit-based academic course of study.

It is just not possible to identify specific competencies that will be expected of you in your practice area. These will entirely depend on the specific requirements of your role. For example, depending on your role you may need to demonstrate competency in the following areas:

- intravenous cannulation;
- interpretation of ECG;
- use of specific syringe drivers;
- defibrillation;
- preparing case notes for court cases;
- leading a case conference;
- undertaking an unsupervised home visit;
- administering chemotherapy;
- use of organisational assessment tools;
- wound care.

Formal assessment

While it is not possible in this book to predict exactly what will be assessed during your preceptorship programme, it should be possible for you to identify specific assessment requirements based on the information you have at your disposal. Firstly, you should be provided with a timetable for your programme which should indicate when formal assessments are likely to take place and also the nature of this assessment (OSCE, observation in practice, online activities or written tests). If your preceptorship programme involves a credit-based academic course, assessment may include some form of written assessment, for example a portfolio or reflective essay. Another way to identify the type of assessment you can expect is to identify the specific knowledge and skills that you may need to fulfil your job description. Refer back to the notes you made in Activity 5.1 to identify what these may be. If there is something specific you are required to do as part of your professional role then you can assume that this will form part of your competency testing. Remember that movement through your KSF gateways will also require some form of assessment or evaluation of your progress.

Informal assessment

Throughout your preceptorship programme you can expect that informal assessment will take place consistently, and through a variety of formats. Typically you will be expected to maintain a post-registration education and practice (PREP) portfolio (Hole, 2009). You can also expect that your PREP portfolio will be reviewed from time to time and feedback given on your progress, typically via your preceptor and /or facilitator of the preceptorship programme.

You will also be required to undertake some form of performance review during your first year after qualification. This may be termed an individual performance review or appraisal. These are typically undertaken by line managers and involve a discussion on areas you would like to develop with constructive feedback related to your performance (Hole, 2009). Both of these methods of informal assessment have one vital thing in common: they both allow you to identify areas that require improvement, and guidance on what may be required to develop your practice.

Using experiential learning to increase knowledge and skills

Throughout your preceptorship programme you will identify areas of knowledge and skill that you need to develop. You may identify these through your own self-assessment/self-awareness, through reflection, feedback or assessment. Regardless of how your learning needs are identified, you must take action to improve the area of knowledge or skill that is lacking. You will need an action plan. In the last chapter we identified the need to set SMART goals and identify resources available to you. We briefly discussed that an experiential cycle can be used to promote acquisition of knowledge and skills.

Kolb's experiential learning cycle

In Chapter 4 we established that Kolb's experiential learning cycle allows a learner to engage with a purposeful and realistic way to learn in, from and during the experiences that formulate daily work. The four stages of Kolb's experiential learning cycle are as follows (see Figure 4.1):

* concrete experience – an immediate experience that forms the basis of observation and feedback;
* reflective observation – critical reflection;
* abstract conceptualisation – abstract concepts and implications of action;
* active experimentation – goal-directed action and evaluation of the consequences (adapted from Light et al., 2009).

The main benefit of Kolb's experiential learning cycle is that it allows for acquisition and reinforcement of knowledge and skills within a nursing context. To understand this we need to look at each stage of the cycle in greater detail.

Concrete experience

Once you have developed a SMART goal you will probably enter the experiential learning cycle at the concrete experience stage; essentially where there is an opportunity to undertake a practice activity (Dennison and Kirk, 1990). Learning in this context occurs when you are able to make links between the experience itself and your learning goal (Cantor, 1995). For example, if you wish to develop your confidence in communicating within team meetings then you might choose a weekly multidisciplinary case review meeting as your concrete experience. If you have identified SMART goals you should be able to make clear links between events in practice and your development requirements. Learning takes place during a concrete experience via 'reflection-in-action' (Schon, 1983), a method of reviewing past experiences, individual values, opinions and expectations in order to learn within the experience (Pattison et al., 2000).

Reflective observation

The second stage in Kolb's experiential learning cycle is an opportunity to reflect on and observe the concrete experience you have had from many perspectives (Kolb, 1984). Termed reflection-on-action (Schon, 1983), this reflection must be guided so that thinking and practice can be moved forward. Ghaye and Lillyman (2000) suggest that a reflective conversation should occur following a reflection-in-action event. In the context of your preceptorship programme this reflective conversation could take place with your preceptor, programme facilitator, peer or line manager. For example, you may reflect on your communication skills following the team meeting, perhaps using feedback from your preceptor to review your performance. Through reflection and feedback it may become clear that your confidence in communicating is hindered by insufficient knowledge related to the care plans of your clients.

Abstract conceptualisation

The abstract conceptualisation stage of the experiential learning cycle relates to the new awareness or knowledge that you will attain following reflection, feedback and further enquiry such as reading policies, research, etc. Learning of new knowledge and skill will take place when you can link current experiences with past experiences, integrate the current experience into what you currently know and test for validity (Boud and Walker, 1993). During this stage of the learning cycle you may be able to identify your specific strengths and weaknesses, or gaps in your knowledge that need to be addressed (Sharples, 2009). For example, if you do recognise a deficit in your knowledge base that is affecting your confidence in communication you could use the abstract conceptualisation stage to develop this area. You might choose to take a more active role in care planning, through liaising with members of the multidisciplinary team and reviewing your care planning technique with senior nurses. You might also choose to review a sample of detailed care plans to identify areas that you could improve on. Learning takes place as a result of abstract conceptualisation because you are able to create concepts that integrate your observations into logically sound theories (Kolb, 1984).

Active experimentation

The last stage of Kolb's experiential learning cycle is the application stage of the cycle where the emphasis is on practical applications as opposed to reflective understanding; there is a pragmatic concern with what works, on influencing people and changing situations (Kolb, 1994). The focus of active experimentation is the application of knowledge and skill. You experience an event, reflect on that event to make sense of what happened and then you adjust your practices as a result of what you have learned. Dennison and Kirk (1990) propose that if the learning cycle up to this point has been successful you will have the capacity and understanding to act differently. At the completion of each learning cycle you should be capable of behaving in a way that you would not have known previously or did not know about when you are next confronted with a new situation (Dennison and Kirk, 1990). For example, your improved knowledge relating to the care needs of your patients could improve your confidence in communicating during team meetings. You could use a subsequent case review meeting to use your improved knowledge to provide a confident and detailed presentation on the progress of your clients. Your experiences of moving through one cycle will naturally lead to additional concrete experiences that will start another cycle all over again (Sharples, 2009).

Activity 5.2: Critical thinking

The experiential learning cycle in action

For this activity we will return to the example of medicines management used previously in the chapter. We will assume that as a newly registered nurse you are required to demonstrate competence in relation to calculation of intravenous infusions. The SMART goal you have set yourself is as follows: *I will accurately calculate the correct dose and infusion rate for continuous insulin infusion.*

The activity requires you to plan how to achieve this goal using an experiential learning cycle. Some prompt questions have been included at each stage to get you started. An outline answer is also provided at the end of this chapter.

> Concrete experience: What type of practice event might provide an opportunity to set up an insulin infusion?

> Reflective observation: What aspect of your competence might you reflect on after the event? Who will you reflect with?

> Abstract conceptualisation: What knowledge or skill may you need to review your practice?

> Active experimentation: How will you know that you are competent? What will you need to do?

There is a brief outline answer to this activity at the end of the chapter.

Peer review and clinical supervision

Throughout your career as a registered nurse you will be exposed to many opportunities for what is known as peer review or clinical supervision. The first thing to clarify is that peer review or clinical supervision is not another term for your appraisal, counselling or having someone look over your shoulder (NHS East of England, 2007). It is simply a means to identify solutions to problems, improve practice and increase awareness of professional issues (Fowler, 1998). It may be undertaken on a one-to-one basis or as a reflective group exercise. During your preceptorship programme you will be expected to take an active role in peer review and clinical supervision. Not only will you learn through the experience of others, but also they in turn will learn through your experiences. The real benefit of peer review or clinical supervision is that it allows for a formalised reflective framework to be incorporated into an experiential learning cycle, typically at the reflective observation and abstract conceptualisation stage (Kolb, 1994). By taking advantage of peer review/clinical supervision you will gain addition insight into your own professional development needs and increase your range of knowledge and skills.

Chapter summary

Throughout this chapter we have discussed the opportunities to increase knowledge and skills through formal and informal assessment during the preceptorship programme. We have reviewed the various types of assessment that you may encounter, the purpose of these assessments and also discussed specific preparation for competency testing. There has been opportunity to discuss the stages of an experiential learning cycle and how these may be implemented to achieve your development goals. Finally we have also explored the links between peer review/clinical supervision and development of knowledge and skills.

Activities: brief outline answers

Activity 5.1: Reviewing specific knowledge and skills (page 47)

This activity required you to review some specific areas of knowledge and skill that you were exposed to during your practice experiences, and also some experiences that you have not been exposed to but will form part of your current role. You may have reviewed a clinical skills profile or similar documentation to record your answer. Some examples are provided below:

- I have achieved competence in aseptic technique. I have never had an opportunity of doing an aseptic dressing for a deep tissue pressure ulcer.
- I have performed a female catheterisation in a simulated experience; I have never performed a catheterisation on a female.
- I have learnt a variety of bandaging techniques. I have not learnt four layer compression bandaging.

Activity 5.2: The experiential learning cycle in action (page 52)

For this activity you were required to plan how to achieve a specific goal using an experiential learning cycle, with the goal: *I will accurately calculate the correct dose and infusion rate for continuous insulin infusion.*

Concrete experience: What type of practice event might provide an opportunity to set up an insulin infusion?

At least two patients every day on my ward are prescribed continuous insulin infusions. I could ensure that I am allocated these patients so I can gain experience in this learning experience.

Reflective observation: What aspect of your competence might you reflect on after the event? Who will you reflect with?

I will reflect on the accuracy of my drug calculation, my skills of preparing the infusion, my knowledge of how to decide on the correct rate of infusion based on the sliding scale and my ability to programme/operate the infusion pump. I will reflect on all these areas with my preceptor and other qualified staff.

Abstract conceptualisation: What knowledge or skill may you need to review or practice?

Depending on the outcome of my reflection I may need to review the following:
- *my skills of preparing the infusion;*
- *the local policy for insulin infusions;*
- *my knowledge of how to decide on the correct rate of infusion;*
- *my ability to programme/operate the infusion pump.*

Active experimentation: How will you know that you are competent? What will you need to do?

In order to be competent I will need to demonstrate the following:
- *accurate preparation of the infusion without prompts or assistance;*
- *accurate interpretation of the sliding scale prescription to ensure the correct rate of infusion;*
- *correct programming/operation of the infusion pump.*

I will need to demonstrate this on multiple occasions to ensure that I can consistently maintain this competency.

Further reading

Fowler, J (1998) *The Handbook of Clinical Supervision – Your Questions Answered.* Salisbury: Quay Books. This easy-to-read text provides an excellent overview of clinical supervision and the value of peer review for ongoing professional development.

Useful websites

The 2010 version of the NMC PREP handbook can be accessed at: **www.nmc-uk.org/Documents/Standards/nmcPrepHandbook.pdf**

If you would like to develop skills related to assessment you could undertake the 'How does my team assess patients?' activity on the Flying Start England website. You can access this activity at: **www.flyingstartengland.nhs.uk/clinical-skills/assessmentandplanning**

If you would like to develop skills related to operation of unfamiliar equipment you may like to undertake the 'Orientation to equipment' activity on the Flying Start NHS website. You can access this activity at: **www.flyingstart.scot.nhs.uk/learning-programmes/clinical-skills/clinical-skills-development.aspx**

Chapter 6
Confidence in applying evidence-based practice

Preceptorship Framework and KSF

This chapter maps to the following elements of the Department of Health Preceptorship Framework and the NHS Knowledge and Skills Framework.

Preceptorship Framework
- Confidence in applying evidence-based practice
- Increase knowledge and clinical skills
- Integrate prior learning into practice
- Team-working

NHS Knowledge and Skills Framework
- Communication
- Personal and people development
- Service improvement
- Quality

Chapter aims

The aim of this chapter is to consider the role of the registered nurse in relation to identifying and implementing evidence-based practice. By the end of this chapter you will be able to:
- understand the importance of applying research to nursing practice;
- identify strategies for implementing evidence-based practice;
- explore practical ways to keep yourself up to date.

Introduction: achieving evidence-based practice

Stop for a moment and consider what it means to be a registered nurse. For many years now you have been studying and aiming for this achievement, and no doubt it was a great relief to finally succeed. All those years of study; all those hours of sacrifice will now feel worth the effort. Yet you have not come this far simply because of what you are capable of doing. While it is true that a significant part of your pre-registration course will have been concerned with a variety of practical skills, the fact is that it is not those skills alone that identify you as a nurse. If a skill set were the only requirement then an intensive course of technical skills over several weeks would no doubt have sufficed. A skilled robot could do the work. The reason that you are a registered nurse is largely a result of proving that you are capable of knowing what it is that you are doing, why you are doing it and are capable of considering alternative approaches based on sound evidence. You are a registered nurse because you are capable of achieving evidence-based practice.

Applying evidence-based practice

One of the many challenges of being a newly registered nurse is in understanding how to apply your theoretical knowledge into daily practice. As a student there was always a safety net when it came to decision-making, either in the form of a mentor or lecturer whose role in part was to discuss and debate decisions and the consequences of actions. You were possibly never really left in a position where it was possible to make a mistake in patient care as so many people were accountable for your actions. As a consequence you will have only proven that you are capable of making decisions based on available evidence, as you could never be left to actually make patient care decisions entirely on your own. Schoessler and Waldo (2006) suggest that once qualified and the immediate transition from student to qualified nurse has taken place, most nurses enter a neutral phase, where the rules of being a student no longer apply but where the rules of the healthcare setting have not yet been mastered. If this feeling is very familiar then don't let this worry you – in fact, you are experiencing a very normal reaction to being a qualified nurse. What may surprise you is that the majority of the discomfort you feel in this stage is due to the uncertainty you have in applying evidence-based practice.

> ### Case study: Steven talks about his transition from student to registered nurse
>
> *My last practice placement that I did before I qualified was in the unit where I got my first job. During my last placement I remember being so confident and feeling in control. Every day I would have a discussion with my mentor about the patients I would be caring for and we would do our care planning together. We used to have all these conversations about how they were progressing with treatment and what the focus of the rehab sessions would be. When I think about it now I think I must have been in a bubble during those weeks because as soon as I was qualified, well that was when reality struck. Every day I would come in and it was like a different world; it was rush, rush, and it seemed like no one had time to talk things through any more. At first I thought it was me; that somehow they didn't like me or something. I spoke to my preceptor and she was really kind, I guess she's had lots of experience with the newly qualified nurses. She just explained that I'm expected to stand on my own two feet now; I'm allowed to make decisions and plan care based on my own knowledge. It came as a shock to be honest that I'm trusted to be making these decisions about care without anyone checking on me all the time. But that's what being a nurse is, I guess, caring for people based on your knowledge and skills. I can remember feeling so confused at the time, proud that I was being trusted to deliver safe care and really scared that I wouldn't have enough knowledge. I know they kept saying at uni that we would need to apply knowledge to practice but it doesn't really sink in until it's you alone with your knowledge.*

In the case study above Steven described difficulties in making his transition because he was lacking confidence in making clinical decisions based on his own knowledge and skills. In other words, he was struggling with the application of evidence-based practice. Steven is certainly not alone in his feelings. Mooney (2006) reports that newly qualified nurses have multiple concerns related to implementing evidence-based practice, including unexpected responsibility, concerns for patient safety and an inability to incorporate theory and practice. If you are experiencing these feelings then the first step is to acknowledge that you are normal. You are simply experiencing the same reaction and fears as many nurses before you and no doubt many newly qualified nurses after you. The next step is to put a new plan in place for learning the new rules of applying evidence-based practice. Remember that the point of registration is only the beginning of a lifelong learning experience and the development of expertise in the role of a registered nurse (Holland et al., 2010).

Applying research to nursing practice

Throughout your pre-registration programme you will have been constantly exposed to a myriad of research and research-based evidence to support nursing practice. In fact, such has been your exposure to research that you may have felt that too much emphasis was placed on it, and struggled at times to see the relevance in your own nursing practice (Hek and Shaw, 2006). In addition, you may feel that research is something that you undertake in a formal sense later in your nursing career, but not particularly relevant at this stage of your preceptorship programme. In truth, however, all of your nursing practice, all aspects of care that you deliver will be (or should be) grounded in research. It is this grounding of research within your day-to-day practice that has given rise to the term 'evidence-based practice'. It refers to the process that you will use to systematically find, appraise and use research findings as the basis of your clinical decisions (Rosenberg and Donald, 1995).

Activity 6.1: Evidence-based practice and research

Audit of evidence-based practice

This activity involves you auditing the scope of evidence-based practice in your practice area. Pick a day at random and ask all registered nurses on that shift to discuss the link between research and one aspect of the care that is routinely delivered. You may choose to do this in a group setting, perhaps a unit meeting. For example, you may ask your colleagues about the evidence base for a nursing procedure such as choice of wound dressings. Alternatively you could ask about the evidence base for a policy such as for visiting hours or meal distribution. Take some time to discuss where this evidence comes from and how the research that supports this practice is disseminated to all staff. Is evidence-based practice regularly discussed in your practice area? Write down some brief notes regarding the information you uncover. We will return to the results of this activity later in the chapter.

There is no answer to this activity as your response will be individual to you.

The importance of evidence-based practice

While the concept of evidence-based practice is certainly not new, it is also clear that its popularity continues to grow year by year. The reason for this is two-fold. Firstly, the rapid flow of information around the world has had a dramatic effect on the application of research, meaning we can all access information far more readily. Harmer (2005) argues that solutions, outcomes and choices for patients now represent the best knowledge available internationally rather than the knowledge of the ward next door. In fact, such is the availability and accessibility to research evidence that service users are seeking out the evidence base for the care being provided and will speak knowledgably about the research base for nursing care. As a newly qualified nurse you may find it quite daunting that the care you deliver is subject to appraisal not just by your peers but also by patients and relatives. As a student you may have been able to effectively 'hide' at times, perhaps relying on the fact that you couldn't always be expected to know. As a qualified practitioner that luxury has effectively been removed; you are expected to know the reasons for your practice, and without this knowledge your practice could be called into question.

Case study: Eunice discusses a patient care episode

I had been qualified about two months and was just starting to find my feet on the ward. I had a lovely patient who had suffered a stroke and he was still requiring enteral feeding. One day his daughter was there while I was cleaning his PEG site and started asking me about my aseptic technique. She had been on the internet and started quoting all these studies from a hospital in America where they had looked at the rationale for daily dressings versus twice daily dressings and whether this increased potential for infection. I tried to bluff but it became clear that I didn't know what she was talking about and I must have been the colour of beetroot. It became clear to both of us that she knew more about best practice for PEG dressings than I did, and yet I was the one meant to be a professional. I remember going home and reading everything I could about the dressings and even got the other staff on the ward looking at the research. It turned out that we were following best practice as this wasn't a new issue and our protocols had been updated only recently. It made an impact on me though. I realised that I had been trying so hard to adjust to being qualified that I forgot how important it was to be able to rationalise everything I was doing. Evidence-based practice is about doing the best for the patient, not just completing tasks because there is work that needs to be done.

Another reason that evidence-based practice continues to predominate nursing practice is the changing and extending role of the nurse. The implementation of the NHS Plan (Department of Health, 2000) and extended nurse prescribing (Department of Health, 2002) has seen nurses take far more responsibility in terms of admitting and discharging patients and also prescribing medications. These roles have meant that nurses are expected to be able to make advanced clinical decisions based on a sound understanding of the available evidence (Banning, 2005).

Strategies for implementing evidence-based practice

One of the major concerns with turning research into evidence-based practice is the time delay between the research taking place, publication, dissemination and implementation. There is a famous example that relates to the difficulty in research being used to change practice. Doreen Norton was a ward sister who undertook research on pressure ulcers. Sadly she found that much of what she uncovered during her research was not new information at all; it simply had not been passed on to inform nursing practice or teaching (Norton, 1988). This may be due to the fact that while most nurses recognise what evidence-based practice is and are familiar with research, they remain unclear regarding how it is to be applied to clinical decision-making (Banning, 2005).

Research summary: NHS Evidence

What is NHS Evidence?

NHS Evidence is a website that was launched in 2009 to manage the synthesis and spread of knowledge in the NHS. Its introduction has ensured that everyone working in health and social care has free access to the quality-assured, best-practice information required to inform evidence-based decision-making, quickly and easily. On NHS Evidence users can search more than 150 sources simultaneously, including internationally respected evidence-based sources such as the Cochrane Library, British National Formulary and Map of Medicine. The types of resources available include guidelines, drug information, primary research and clinical summaries. NHS Athens account holders can also get free access to paid-for databases of evidence, e-books and key journals.

Specialist collections

In addition to providing web, medical database, journal and e-book searches, NHS Evidence is also home to more than 30 digital specialist collections, which provide annual evidence updates on key areas, giving a straightforward and succinct overview of what new research and evidence has been published.

QIPP: Quality, Innovation, Productivity and Prevention

The QIPP collection is designed to help the NHS meet its current challenges of addressing inefficiencies while also improving patient care. It brings together practical examples of how NHS organisations are improving quality whilst making efficiency savings. It allows colleagues across the NHS to share best practice and deliver successful improvements without having to 're-invent the wheel'. Examples range from one-off studies from single organisations to robustly tested large-scale changes that have been replicated in multiple organisations with results published in academic journals. The aim is to build a comprehensive base of best practice examples that others can learn from.

NHS Evidence can be found at: **www.evidence.nhs.uk**.

Professional implications for evidence-based practice

It is clear that nurses may find it difficult to make direct links between research and their practice; however, from a professional perspective this has vast implications. The requirement to embed evidence-based practice into care of patients is clearly outlined within the NMC Code of Conduct. Specifically you are required to:

- deliver care based on the best available evidence or best practice;
- ensure any advice you give is evidence-based if you are suggesting healthcare products or services (NMC, 2008a).

Likewise, the *PREP Handbook* (NMC, 2008b) clearly indicates that learning activities relevant to your area of practice must be undertaken and recorded as evidence for renewal of registration (Hole, 2009). In addition, you will need a clear understanding of the value of the research in terms of its significance and usefulness to your practice (Bircumshaw, 1990). The fact that you have just completed your pre-registration education should put you at an advantage here, as you should have a current knowledge of research teaching and understanding of the research process (Hek and Shaw, 2006). You should be well versed in being able to judge the rigour of research evidence and its applicability to your practice (Humphris, 2005). From now on and for the remainder of your nursing career you will rely on this knowledge to justify your professional qualification. As a registered nurse you must be able to demonstrate that you are able to critically question evidence that is presented in order to make an informed judgement about its robustness and utility to your practice (LoBiondo-Wood, 1990).

Evidence-based practice in practice

Perhaps the biggest challenge facing nurses when it comes to evidence-based practice is bridging the gap between finding the evidence and implementing it in practice. While there may be a general willingness amongst nurses to follow the principles of evidence-based practice, the implementation often requires a forum that is either not readily available or not readily accessible. There are a number of key reasons as to why nurses may not always embed evidence-based practice into their care. These include:

- not making the effort to keep up to date;
- being comfortable with traditional or ritual practices;
- lacking resources (e.g. time) to seek out the evidence;
- lacking confidence to change;
- restrictions within the organisation (Joyce, 2005).

While these issues are real and can often be problematic, this does not mean that there are no solutions or alternatives that can be utilised to offset these barriers.

Overcoming barriers to evidence-based practice

One of the easiest approaches you can take to evidence-based practice is to assume the responsibility for keeping yourself up to date regarding current research in your speciality. Once you have identified a specialty area seek out a quality research journal that publishes within this area. You could consider subscribing to the journal to ensure you receive regular updates, or accessing the journal online or in a local library. Just taking the time to read one or two articles per month will help you remain current in your field of practice. Encourage others to do the same by placing relevant articles on notice boards or in research folders (Hek and Shaw, 2005).

Access to resources

While refereed journals are a valuable resource for accessing research, they are by no means the only source. The process of embedding evidence-based practice has many facets, and it is generally up to the individual to find a method that is suitable. It has become quite popular to discuss research and evidence-based practice within staff meetings, either locally or as an organisation-wide clinical governance event. Staff meetings are excellent opportunities to discuss care and ensure a consistent approach is maintained. You could even consider using the results of Activity 6.1 you undertook previously in the chapter and ask to discuss this at your next staff meeting. Whatever approach you take, remember that every time you actively engage with evidence-based practice you are aiming to ensure that every patient receives the best possible care (Klardie et al., 2004).

Activity 6.2: Evidence-based practice and research

Opportunities for evidence-based practice

Depending on your organisation you may have access to a number of opportunities for engaging with evidence-based practice. Use the grid below to identify the opportunities currently available to you, and also how you may become involved in these areas.

Evidence-based practice activities	Opportunities to become involved
Project work	
Auditing	
Notice boards	
Teaching of students and/or other staff	

continued overleaf...

continued...

Evidence-based practice activities	Opportunities to become involved
Internet searches	
Library access	
Journal clubs	
Staff meetings	

There is a brief outline answer to this activity at the end of the chapter.

While you may be provided with an opportunity of undertaking the activities represented in Activity 6.2 during work time, you should not restrict your evidence-based activity to time that is sanctioned by the organisation. Just like your study activity, remaining clinically current is a part of your professional role, and this will make demands on your own time (Hek and Shaw, 2005).

Chapter summary

Throughout this chapter we have looked at the role of the registered nurse in relation to identifying and implementing evidence-based practice. We have identified that research provides the foundation for applying a strong evidence base for nursing practice. There has also been an opportunity to identify strategies for implementing evidence-based practice and suggestions for overcoming barriers. This has included practical ways to keep yourself and your practice up to date. We will be returning to evidence-based practice throughout this book, particularly in relation to audit (Chapter 10) and management of risk (Chapter 13). Of course, the confidence to apply many of these techniques will be somewhat dependent on your interpersonal skills, which we will address in Chapter 9.

Activities: brief outline answer

Activity 6.2: Opportunities for evidence-based practice (page 61)

This activity required you to identify the opportunities currently available for specific evidence-based practice activities. A sample of how this may look is provided.

Evidence-based practice activities	Opportunities to become involved
Project work	*No specific project.*
Auditing	*Monthly audit of key performance indicators – I could become involved in audit of handwashing.*
Notice boards	*There is a staff research notice board. I could put up research article of interest.*
Teaching of students and/or other staff	*No specific opportunities.*
Internet searches	*My Trust has internet access for staff. I should contact IT and get my own username and password.*
Library access	*My Trust has a large library. I can access journals for my specialty there free of charge.*
Journal clubs	*No club running at present but I could start one.*
Staff meetings	*There is a staff meeting every week. I could discuss any new research I read about in the staff meeting.*

Further reading

Harmer, S and Collinson, G (2005) *Achieving Evidence based Practice*, 2nd edn. London: Balliere Tindall. This book provides a comprehensive and easy-to-follow guide to evidence-based practice. With practical examples and reflective activities, this book addresses all aspects of evidence-based practice in nursing.

Useful websites

www.nice.org.uk/
The website of the National Institute of Health and Clinical Excellence. NHS Evidence users can search more than 150 sources simultaneously, including internationally respected evidence-based sources such as the Cochrane Library, British National Formulary and Map of Medicine. The types of resources available include guidelines, drug information, primary research and clinical summaries. NHS Athens account holders can also get free access to paid-for databases of evidence, e-books and key journals.

If you would like to develop your skills for undertaking a literature search you may find the 'Top tips for literature searching' activity on the Flying Start NHS website useful. You can access this activity at: **www.flyingstart.scot.nhs.uk/learning-programmes/research-for-practice/ research-literacy.aspx**

If you would like to look at a specific area of evidence-based practice you may find the 'Evidence based practice model' activity a useful way of undertaking this. You can access this resource at: **www.flyingstartengland.nhs.uk/researchforpractice/evidencebasedpractice**

Chapter 7
Understanding policies and procedures

Preceptorship Framework and KSF

This chapter maps to the following elements of the Department of Health Preceptorship Framework and the NHS Knowledge and Skills Framework.

Preceptorship Framework
- Understand policies and procedures
- Confidence in applying evidence-based practice
- Implement the Code and professional values
- Integrate prior learning into practice
- Managing risk and not being risk averse

NHS Knowledge and Skills Framework
- Health, safety and security
- Service improvement
- Quality

Chapter aims

The aim of this chapter is to explore the importance of understanding policies and procedures and your own accountability and responsibility in relation to them. It is recommended that this chapter should be read in conjunction with Chapter 13 on managing risk. By the end of this chapter you will be able to:

- appreciate your own responsibility and accountability with regard to implementing and following policies and procedures;
- understand how policies are developed both within your organisation and nationally, and how to access them;
- apply local policies and procedures within your practice to deliver safe and effective care.

Why are policies and procedures required?

Evidence-based policies, procedures and protocols are essential to ensure high quality clinical standards. In law there is no hierarchy between them but each of them should be followed where reasonably possible (Dimond, 2008). Other terms you may hear used are guidelines, standards, patient group directions and care bundles; each of these terms are defined in Table 7.1 but for ease of reading we will use the term policy to cover all these terms.

Policy	A statement of intent or plan of action. Will outline specific details or rules that must be met.
Procedure	A step-by-step action plan that may or may not be attached to a policy. Written so that everyone undertakes the procedure in an agreed and consistent manner to achieve a safe and effective outcome.
Guideline	A statement of good practice, principles giving practical guidance, allowing for professional initiative. Used to inform decision-making.
Protocol	Detailed descriptions of the steps taken to deliver care or treatment to a patient.
Patient group directions	A written direction that enables supply and administration of medicines to specific groups of patients by specific groups of professionals without a prescription.
Standards	Specific statements of desired performance which are definable and achievable.
Care bundles	A group of evidence-based interventions related to a disease or care process that, when executed together, result in better outcomes than when implemented individually (NPSA, 2009).

Table 7.1: Definitions

Activity 7.1: Evidence-based practice and research

How to find local policies

Find out where and how to access your organisation's policies and procedures. Look at the list of policies and procedures available and identify those that you feel have immediate relevance to you.

There is a brief outline answer to this activity at the end of the chapter.

The organisation you work for will have a range of policies; in fact, the larger the organisation the greater number of these documents they are likely to have in place! They are developed to provide rules or guidance to enable employees to deliver outcomes that are consistent and reliable. Some policies will be developed in response to legal requirements; for example, the Health and Safety at Work Act (1994) and the Equality Act (2010), which encompasses many separate Acts such as the Disability Discrimination Act (1995). These policies will influence policies regarding moving and handling and recruitment and selection, for example. Other policies will be based on research or best evidence or on guidelines from organisations such as the National Institute for Health and Clinical Excellence (NICE) and the Royal Colleges, which develop clinical guidelines and standards for healthcare. Policies play a crucial role in risk management and protect not only patients and clients but also visitors and staff. Chapter 13 looks at risk management in more detail.

Case study: Jasmine on the drug round

Jasmine has been in post for four months. It has been a really busy morning. Whilst doing the lunchtime drug round the theatre porters arrive for one of her patients. She has just given Mr Jones his drugs but he is very slow in taking them so she leaves the medicine pot on his bedside locker and locks the drug trolley whilst she deals with the patient for theatre. When she returns to her drug round Mr Jones says that he had taken some but then dropped his medicine pot on the floor. Jasmine cannot see any of the tablets on the floor but Mr Jones explains that the ward domestic assistant had just swept the floor. Jasmine realises that she now has no idea as to which drugs Mr Jones has taken as Mr Jones has poor eyesight and is unclear as to which he has already taken.

In this scenario Jasmine failed to follow the policy for the administration of drugs, which requires the nurse to observe the patient actually taking their drugs. To have avoided this situation Jasmine should have either waited until the patient had taken all his tablets, or locked the tablets away until she could return and observe him taking them all.

Interruptions on drug rounds have been shown to be significantly associated with medication errors (Westbrook et al., 2010) which has led some hospitals to require nurses to wear distinctive tabards or vests, although there is at present inconclusive evidence that these reduce the level of interruptions (Scott et al., 2010) and more evidence is required to develop strategies to reduce interruptions.

Research summary: medication errors

Incorrect administration of medication (which often occurs due to failures to follow the drug administration policy) was the second most common allegation referred to the NMC's conduct and competence committee in 2008–9 (10.75% of all cases) (NMC, 2009b) and medication incidents were the third largest group (9%) of all incidents reported to the National Patient Safety Agency's (NPSA) Reporting and Learning System (RLS) in 2007. A review of patient safety for children and young people by the NPSA published in 2009 reported that the most commonly reported incident type for children (17% of all cases) related to medication incidents, particularly in the 0–4 years age group (NPSA, 2009). The most likely cause of these incidents is the complexity of dose calculation and the fact that children in neonatal units receive a larger number of medications than other groups of children. The NPSA website reports that the most common causes of medication errors reported to them relate to:
- wrong dose;
- omitted or delayed medicines;
- wrong medicine.

In each case procedural errors will have taken place including failure to follow policy with regard to the administration of medicines.

How policies are developed

Most organisations will have a corporate approach to ensure that all their policies are developed in the same way and follow the same format, distribution and review processes. All policies must be mindful of the Equality Act (2010). The trigger to develop a new policy may arise from a number of sources:

- new guidance on an aspect of healthcare practice or treatment, e.g. a new National Service Framework, NICE Clinical Guideline, NMC Standard or Guidance publication;
- a response to major incidents or significant failure(s) in care locally or nationally, e.g. a review of safeguarding policies and procedures by organisations following the death of Baby P in Haringey in 2008 (The Lord Lamming, 2009), new policies developed for the management of *Clostridium difficile* after outbreaks in a number of acute Trusts, which led to investigations between 2006 and 2007 (Healthcare Commission, 2006, 2007);
- the introduction of a new policy by the government, e.g. the Disability Discrimination Act 2005 placed a general and specific duty on public authorities to promote disability equality and to eliminate institutional disability discrimination.

A designated lead person will be identified to develop a new policy (or review a current one) in consultation with key reference groups which will include experts in the area of policy being developed. Policies that guide practice must be evidence-based and national guidance should be used where published. The key areas a policy is likely to cover are:

- title (making clear whether a policy, standard, guideline, etc.);
- date written;
- introduction/purpose/aim;
- background/relevant legislation/national guidance/evidence base;
- scope of policy;
- definitions;
- policy/procedure main body;
- roles and responsibilities;
- education and development;
- risk assessment;
- monitoring and review (including date for review);
- references/evidence.

Once written, all policies should have an equality impact assessment undertaken to ensure that they do not disadvantage any groups. The policy should then go to consultation with key stakeholders before being ratified by the organisation's board or a group of individuals who have that delegated authority. All policies must be indexed and easily accessible to all staff and in most cases made available on either the organisation's internet or the intranet site.

Keeping up to date

Trying to keep up-to-date with current policies and procedures can be challenging. All staff should be informed of any new policies developed by their employing organisation that are relevant to them. In addition, it is important to be aware of what is happening outside the organisation you work for. As discussed earlier there are a number of organisations that develop standards, guidance and tools which influence the development of policies at a local level. These organisations and the publications they produce are a valuable resource to enable you to read up on best evidence for practice and identify new evidence that you may wish to use to introduce new policies or update current ones.

National Institute for Health and Clinical Excellence (NICE)

NICE provides evidence-based standards and clinical guidelines relating to a wide range of health conditions. The clinical guidelines bring together the most up-to-date clinical evidence for treating and managing a specific condition, taking into account the cost-effectiveness of different approaches. They are based on the whole patient journey from diagnosis to treatment, although short guidelines are developed which cover only one part of the care pathway where there is an urgent demand for advice in a specific area.

High impact interventions for nursing and midwifery

The high impact interventions are examples from nurses and midwives who have implemented simple changes that have made differences in patient safety, the quality of care and the patient experience, as well as improving the experience for nurses and midwives in caring for patients and clients and reducing costs. Following a request by the Chief Nursing Officer for England for nurses and midwives to submit examples of high impact interventions, eight interventions were selected and published covering:

- reducing falls;
- improving nutrition;
- reducing pressure ulcers;
- promoting normal birth;
- increasing patient choice about where to die;
- reducing sickness and absence;
- nursing- and midwifery-led discharges;
- reduction in urinary tract infections (UTIs) (NHS Institute for Innovation and Improvement, 2009).

In addition, there are over 500 other examples on the NHS Institute for Innovation and Improvement's website (**www.institute.nhs.uk**), which cover a range of interventions relevant to different fields of practice.

National Clinical Guideline Centre (NCGC)

This centre produces evidence-based clinical practice guidelines on behalf of NICE and is overseen by the Royal Colleges of General Practitioners, Nursing, Physicians and Surgeons. A range of guidelines are listed with links to NICE and the Royal College of Nursing for additional tools to aid their implementation.

NHS Evidence Health Information Resources

This website brings together links to a range of other websites as well as access to a range of resources that will enable you to search for best evidence and information, including:

- National Library of Guidelines, a range of guidelines for the NHS from over 100 organisations;
- NHS Clinical Knowledge Summaries, which are aimed at healthcare professionals working in primary care and first contact care and which provide evidence-based information for managing common conditions seen in primary care;
- evidence-based reviews, e.g. Cochrane database;
- journals and healthcare databases;
- drugs information, e.g. *British National Formulary*;
- information sites for patients accredited by NHS Direct online.

Activity 7.2: Evidence-based practice and research

National policies, procedures and guidelines

Go to the National Clinical Guideline Centre (NCGC) website at: **www.ncgc.ac.uk**; look at their list of clinical guidelines, and identify ones which have direct relevance to the area you work in or the client group you care for. Find out if there are any local policies, procedures or standards that have been developed in response to the guideline/standards you have chosen.

If there are some guidelines or standards on the NICE website that don't have local policies/procedures/standards, consider what your responsibility might be and what you might do about it.

There is a brief outline answer to this activity at the end of the chapter.

Statutory and mandatory training

All organisations will have a number of statutory and mandatory training programmes which staff are required to attend. Many of these will be underpinned by policies and so are a valuable means of ensuring that you are familiar with the key policies in your organisation. Failure to attend sessions could lead to disciplinary action and it is important therefore that you record attendance at all sessions in your professional portfolio.

Statutory training sessions are ones which your employer is required to provide by law and usually applies to all employees; for example, fire training and equality and diversity training.

Mandatory training is training that has been identified by your employer as required to limit risk and to ensure that safe working practice is maintained, and may often be specific to certain roles.

Common statutory and mandatory training sessions for nurses and midwives are detailed in Table 7.2.

Fire training	Equality and diversity	Basic life support/ resuscitation
Child protection	Data protection	Health and safety/ COSHH/Risk/ Incident reporting
Infection control and decontamination	Information governance	Medicines management
Moving and handling	Medical equipment/devices	Protecting vulnerable adults
Blood transfusion	Violence and aggression Conflict resolution	Handling complaints
Slips, trips and falls	Food hygiene	

Table 7.2: Common statutory and mandatory training sessions

Many of the statutory and mandatory sessions will have been included as part of your induction to the organisation you work for, but you will be required to attend further updates for some of them every one to three years depending on your organisation's requirements.

Professional accountability and responsibility

The NMC is very clear in *The Code: Standards of Conduct, Performance and Ethics for Nurses and Midwives* (NMC, 2008a) regarding your personal accountability for your actions and omissions in your practice. They highlight the need to ensure that you use the best available evidence when delivering care. The policies and procedures that you implement on a daily basis will, wherever possible, be based on best evidence and therefore failure to follow local policies could lead not only to your employer taking disciplinary action against you, but also cause them to refer you to the NMC for failing to comply with the Code, as this would raise concerns about your fitness to practise. Clearly, referral to the NMC could endanger your registration. Your employer has a responsibility to ensure that you are offered appropriate education and training and so you will be expected to attend statutory and mandatory training sessions to keep up-to-date with current legislation and local policies. Failing to attend these sessions could mean that you are unaware of changes in policy and could therefore put your patients at risk through incorrect practice, and put your own career at risk for failing to follow best practice. Equally, if education and training are not available to you, the responsibility to make this known is yours, as lack of availability is not an excuse.

Society today is far more litigious; it is therefore imperative that you follow policies, procedures and guidelines, as failure to do so could be seen in law as a breach in the standard of care (Dimond, 2008). It is important to also note that if you are aware that a certain policy is no longer based on best evidence and fail to bring this to the attention of those responsible and continue to follow that policy and a patient comes to harm then you would be deemed to be negligent.

Chapter summary

This chapter has looked at policies and procedures and highlighted why it is important that you are fully conversant with key policies in order to ensure that your patients receive high quality care based on best evidence and are not put at risk through substandard practice. Policies and procedures also provide you with protection; failure to follow them could potentially lead to instigation of the disciplinary process and, should patients come to harm, referral to the NMC.

Activities: Brief outline answers

Activity 7.1: How to find local policies (page 66)

The list of policies and procedures you have found may be quite daunting. Remember that policies are applicable to all employees so all policies will be relevant to you. However, if you want to prioritise which ones to read first, the following are ones that have been suggested by senior colleagues who work in the NHS:

- HR policies;
- medication management;
- falls;
- infection control;
- complaints;
- vulnerable adults;
- safeguarding;
- privacy and dignity;
- equality and diversity.

Activity 7.2: National poicies, procedures and guidelines (page 70)

Your answer to this activity will depend on what policies, procedures, etc., are already in place in your organisation. If you found a clinical guideline that doesn't appear to have a local policy you should discuss this with your manager or lead for clinical governance. If it is something that is applicable to your area but not to the wider organisation, you could work with your colleagues to develop a local policy/guidance document that will guide best practice.

Further reading

Dougherty, L and Lister, S (eds) (2008) *The Royal Marsden Hospital Manual of Clinical Nursing Procedures*, 7th edn. Oxford: Wiley-Blackwell.
This book contains evidence-based information and guidance on a wide range of clinical nursing procedures. Many NHS Trusts have an off-line version available on their website.

Useful websites

A key skill that you will also need to develop is networking. The 'Multiprofessional networks' activity on the Flying Start NHS website would be a useful starting point to explore this approach to working with other healthcare professionals. You will find the details of this activity at: **www.flyingstart.scot.nhs. uk/learning-programmes/policy/understanding-policy.aspx**

To develop your confidence in developing and influencing policy you may find the 'Influencing policy' activity on the Flying Start England website useful to complete. You will find the details of this activity at: **www.flyingstartengland.nhs.uk/policy/influencingpolicy**

National Institute for Health and Clinical Excellence (NICE) website, **www.nice.org.uk**, provides evidence-based standards and clinical guidelines in relation to a wide range of health conditions.

The Royal College of Nursing website, **www.rcn.org.uk**, provides evidence-based standards and clinical guidelines in relation to a wide range of health conditions.

The National Clinical Guideline Centre (NCGC) website, **www.ncgc.ac.uk**, provides evidence-based clinical practice guidelines.

The NHS Evidence Health Information Resources website, **www.library.nhs.uk/**, is a multiresource website of best evidence.

Chapter 8
Team-working

Chapter aims

The aim of this chapter is to explore your role within the multidisciplinary team. By the end of this chapter you will be able to:

- appreciate why teamwork is essential in healthcare;
- identify the key members of the multidisciplinary team;
- appreciate your role and responsibilities within the team;
- identify the challenges of team-working and develop strategies to manage them.

Teamwork

Teamwork has been identified as essential to the effective working of healthcare organisations. The Department of Health's report, *A High Quality Workforce: NHS Next Stage Review* (Department of Health, 2008a), repeatedly makes reference to the importance of the team and the valuable contribution each has to make, be they people in supporting roles, clinicians or managers. In *Modernising Nursing Careers – Setting the Direction*, written by the Chief Nursing Officer's directorate (Department of Health, 2006), the future role of the nurse is seen as one where they will *work as leaders and members of multidisciplinary teams inside and outside hospital, and across health and social care teams* (Department of Health, 2006, page 10).

A number of investigations into failings in patient care have identified that poor teamwork was a contributing factor to the failings (see the Victoria Climbé inquiry (Lamming, 2003), Bristol inquiry (Department of Health, 2001b) and the Mid Staffordshire NHS Foundation Trust inquiry (Francis, 2010)). Each of these inquiries has resulted in recommendations for greater collaborative working.

The importance of working as part of a team is also detailed in the NMC Code (NMC, 2008a), which states that you must *work with others to protect and promote the health and wellbeing of those in your care, their families and carers, and the wider community*, and then in more detail states that in order to work effectively as a team you must:

- work co-operatively within teams and respect the skills, expertise and contributions of your colleagues;
- be willing to share your skills and experience for the benefit of your colleagues;
- consult and take advice from colleagues when appropriate;
- treat your colleagues fairly and without discrimination;
- make a referral to another practitioner when it is in the best interests of someone in your care.

Teamwork can be defined as *a dynamic process involving two or more healthcare professionals with complementary backgrounds and skills, sharing common health goals and exercising concerted physical and mental effort in assessing, planning, or evaluating patient care. This is accomplished through interdependent collaboration, open communication and shared decision-making. This in turn generates value-added patient, organizational and staff outcomes* (Xyrichis and Ream, 2007, page 238).

While the above suggests that teamwork involves two or more healthcare professionals, it is likely that as a newly registered nurse you will be working in an area with a much larger team than two people, although on a day-to-day basis you may work closely with a small number creating a team within a team. For example, you may be a member of a nursing team which is part of a larger nursing team as well as being a member of a multidisciplinary team.

Activity 8.1: Teamwork

Who is in your team?

Use a large sheet of paper to map out in groups all the people who are involved in patient care in your area. Start by identifying groups (e.g. allied health professionals, doctors, social services, support workers, etc.) and then try to put names of individuals where possible.

Identify what you believe to be the key roles and responsibilities of the different team members.

Use circles to show how the different groups overlap in working together to deliver care to your patients/clients.

There is a brief outline answer to this activity at the end of the chapter.

Approaches to team-working

Within the literature references are made to multidisiciplinary, multiprofessional, interprofessional, interdisciplinary and intradisciplinary teams. This can be quite confusing and in many cases they appear to be used interchangeably (Leathard, 2003).

Payne (2000) breaks down the different terms by looking at the different elements that make up each word. 'Multi' means many. In this case a number of different people work separately, each bringing their own specialist expertise to the situation. 'Inter' implies collaborative working between people from different professions or disciplines, with the individuals willing to adapt and adjust their roles, skills and knowledge to work collegiately with their colleagues from other professions or disciplines. 'Intra' is used when a team of people consists of people from the same profession but different specialisms such as mental health nursing, adult nursing, etc.

Based on the above, a patient under the care of a multidisciplinary or multiprofessional team will therefore usually be seen by each member of the team separately, with the team then meeting up at a later point together for a multidisciplinary/professional team meeting to discuss the patient concerned.

In an interprofessional team the team members work together, sharing views and professional knowledge, with possible blurring of the boundaries of their roles. Teams that work interprofessionally will usually put the patient at the centre and they will be actively involved in the discussions that take place. Whichever approach to team-working is used, the focus should always be that the team members are working together for the benefit of the patient or client.

Increasingly nurses are also involved in multi-agency working. Multi-agency working is where different services come together to prevent problems arising in the first place and is commonly seen in relation to vulnerable groups such as children, people with a disability, learning disability or mental illness and the elderly. Multi-agency working can be problematic as it frequently involves professionals from a wide range of agencies including healthcare, social care, education and the independent and voluntary sectors. Consequently there is a move to develop interagency or integrated teams with members based together to improve cross-boundary working.

Activity 8.2: Teamwork

How does your team work?

Review the different members of your team that you identified in Activity 8.1 and consider how they all work together. Which approach to team-working is used? Why do you think that approach is taken?

There is no answer to this activity as it will be personal to you.

The approach used in your workplace will depend on your client group, the professionals involved and where you are based. You may have one team leader co-ordinating the work of the different professional members or each professional may be managed by a team leader from their own professional group.

Benefits of team-working

Borril et al. (2002) suggest that where people work in teams, communication between members of the team and the negotiation that takes place can enable greater clarity of the roles within the team. However, this is only likely to occur if effective communication exists and the members share the same goals.

In their concept analysis of teamwork, Xyrichis and Ream (2007) identified a number of positive outcomes from teamwork, which are shown in Table 8.1.

For **health professionals**	<ul><li>Job satisfaction</li><li>Recognition of individual contribution and motivation</li><li>Improved mental health</li></ul>
For **patients**	<ul><li>Improved quality of care</li><li>Vaue-added patient outcomes</li><li>Satisfaction with services</li></ul>
For **the healthcare organisation**	<ul><li>Satisfied and committed workforce</li><li>Cost control</li><li>Workforce retention and reduced turnover</li></ul>

Table 8.1: Positive outcomes from teamwork

Certainly for you as a newly registered nurse there are significant benefits to working as part of a team, in particular the social, emotional and professional support that colleagues can provide you (Borril et al., 2002), all of which are important given the significant challenges you face as you transition from one role to another.

Barriers and challenges to teamwork

There are a number of barriers and/or challenges that can impact on the effectiveness of team-working. Two major barriers to team-working are a poor understanding of the different roles of the other members of the team and issues around professional boundaries (Atwal and Caldwell, 2006; Cook, 2008).

Pre-registration professional healthcare programmes now include teaching on interprofessional working and many universities now provide shared learning in many of their modules at undergraduate and postgraduate level to encourage greater understanding of the roles and responsibilities of different members of the health and social care team. As part of your preceptorship period it will be helpful for you to spend time with members from the different professional groups who provide care for your client group to enhance your own understanding of their roles.

Professional issues arise from the way different professional groups define their boundaries and work to protect those boundaries when they perceive others encroaching on them (Cook, 2008).

There is an increasing push at government and organisational level to break down professional boundaries within healthcare to provide a more flexible workforce and enhance team-working, but these new ways of working have proved threatening for some who wish to protect their professional identity (Nancarrow and Borthwick, 2005). Professional issues also relate to the different power and status accorded to different professional groups within healthcare, usually with doctors seen as the dominant profession. Atwal and Caldwell (2005) found that doctors dominated multidisciplinary team meetings and that nurses and therapists were less likely to offer opinions and information. This was due in part to the status and hierarchy accorded to the medical profession as well as the gender imbalance that still exists between the medical profession and nursing and therapists.

As a newly registered nurse, while it will be daunting to challenge the views and opinion of others, it is important to remember that you have a responsibility to advocate for the patient and a responsibility to challenge decisions which you do not believe are in their best interest.

Cook (2008) also identified the issue of time and space as a challenge for team-working, which can adversely impact on effective communication between team members. Heavy workloads mean that different professional groups have difficulty in attending meetings; additionally, teams are often located in different areas, further reducing opportunities for contact. Within nursing teams an increasing number of nurses now work 12-hour shifts, which can reduce the opportunities for team members to meet and discuss working practices because there are fewer shift overlaps. It will be important for you to find out how information is shared within your team, not only about the day-to-day care of patients but also information at an organisational and strategic level that impacts on their practice. Are regular team meetings held, and if so how often and when? Is there a communication book or notice board? While you should be informed about communication methods as part of your induction you also have a responsibility to find out this information if it is not offered.

Joining the team

Were you recently a student? If so, your experiences of starting a new placement and the ease or difficulties you experienced in joining the different teams on each placement will be fresh in your mind. However, this time joining the team will be very different because of the change in your role. As a student you were joining what Etienne Wenger calls a community of practice (Wenger, 1998), where the key purpose is one of learning. Your mentor will have facilitated your entry into the team, providing the opportunities for your learning. As a qualified nurse your role will be very different and as a consequence so will the expectations of your colleagues in the team.

Your role within the team

As a new member you will be faced with the challenge of finding your place within the team. The use of grades or bands within nursing promotes the notion of a hierarchy of roles and whilst they may reflect the level of knowledge, skills and experience individuals have, your grade is not the only way to define your place. The research summary on team roles summarises the work undertaken by Dr Meredith Belbin, which identifies the different roles that individuals play as part of a team.

Research summary: team roles

Dr Meredith Belbin undertook a study of teams at Henley Management College in the 1970s in order to determine why some teams are successful whilst others fail. The research, undertaken over ten years, found that the key to successful teams was the balance of different roles within the team. Nine team roles were eventually identified:

- co-ordinator – usually the team leader or chairperson, who guides the group, identifies goals and delegates tasks and activities;
- completer-finisher – ensures the group meets deadlines; is conscientious, with meticulous attention to detail;
- implementer – turns the groups ideas/tasks into practical manageable activities;
- monitor-evaluator – critically analyses ideas and arguments, sees all options and often has a strategic overview;
- plant – the ideas person, comes up with creative, out-of-the-box ideas;
- resource investigator – another ideas person but brings together ideas from a range of sources, a good communicator whose enthusiasm drives the team;
- shaper – pulls ideas together, keeps the team focused and overcomes obstacles;
- specialist – a resource who has specific knowledge and can provide expert advice;
- team-worker – looks after the relationships within the team, who is process-focused, with good collaborative skills (Belbin, 2010).

Depending on the size of the team, individuals may take on more than one of the roles described above. It is quite likely that many of the members will see themselves as specialists as each will have particular knowledge and skills they will bring to the team and the patient or client's care pathway. Nurses play a pivotal role within the multidisciplinary team because they have a close ongoing contact with their patients on a day-to-day basis. They bring their knowledge of the patient as a person and the responses by the patient to the different care interventions to the members of the team.

Consider which roles you take on when working as part of a team and whether any of these roles are missing from the teams you work in. You may find that you have a different role within your nursing team to the one you undertake within the multidisciplinary team.

Team skills

Belbin's work on team roles is helpful in understanding how different members may work within the team; but for a team to work effectively there is also a core of skills that all team members need. These skills fall within the heading of interpersonal skills and are:

- self-awareness;
- communication skills;
- negotiation skills.

Team members need to be aware of how others perceive them and how their own values and beliefs may impact on the way they interact with others. Effective communication is essential; each member needs to be able to state their ideas clearly, listen to the ideas and views of others and use open questioning to enable ideas to be explored and understood. Assertiveness skills would be included here as well. Negotiation skills are also important so that where any disagreements arise, conflict can be avoided. Chapters 9 and 11 explore interpersonal skills and negotiation and conflict resolution further and give you an opportunity to understand your own strengths and scope for development in these areas.

Activity 8.3: Teamwork

Identifying your contribution to the team

Reflect on the feedback you received whilst a student or from previous posts you have held. What were your strengths? What do you feel you can bring to the team?

There is a brief outline answer to this activity at the end of the chapter.

Chapter summary

Effective teamwork has been shown to have positive outcomes for patient care as well as increasing job satisfaction. The knowledge and skills required to work effectively as part of a team include a clear understanding of the roles and responsibilities of the team members and the ability to communicate effectively with each of them. The close, day-to-day contact that nurses have with patients means that they have a pivotal role to play in ensuring that effective communication takes place between the different members of the multidisciplinary team and co-ordinating the care that takes place.

Activities: brief outline answers

Activity 8.1: Who is in your team? (page 75)

Once you have completed this activity check out your diagram with members of your team at work to see if they agree with you and whether you have missed anyone out.

Consider the different roles and responsibilities of each team member. Were there any aspects of their role that you were unaware of? As a nurse you will often be required to co-ordinate the activities of the different team members so having a clear understanding of their roles is essential if patients are to receive care from the most appropriate team members.

Activity 8.3: Identifying your contribution to the team (page 80)

You may have identified a number of ways that you can contribute to the team and the type of team role(s) you feel comfortable with. It is also important to remember that as a new member of the team you will bring a fresh perspective to the team. One of the benefits of a new team member is their ability to identify approaches to care delivery that have become custom and practice but that may no longer be as effective, evidence-based or appropriate. It can be daunting to suggest areas that could be improved, but poor, inefficient or ineffective practice can never be condoned.

Further reading

Goodman, B and Clemow, R (2010) *Nursing and Collaborative Practice: Transforming Nursing Practice*, 2nd edn. Exeter: Learning Matters.

Useful websites

To develop your confidence in working within a team you may find the 'What kind of team player are you?' activity on the Flying Start England website useful to complete. You will find the details of this activity at: **www.flyingstartengland.nhs.uk/teamwork/teamplayers**

To develop your confidence in networking outside your team you may find the 'Multi-professional Networks' activity on the Flying Start NHS website useful to complete. You will find the details of this activity at: **www.flyingstart.scot.nhs.uk/learning-programmes/teamwork/networking.aspx**

The website **www.belbin.com** is Belbin's own website with a range of information and resources around team roles.

Chapter 9
Communication and interpersonal skills

Chapter aims

The aim of this chapter is to explore strategies for developing interpersonal skills and implementing a range of practical communication strategies. By the end of this chapter you will be able to:

- identify the range of communication strategies that will be required within your professional role;
- explore practical techniques for improving your written/verbal communication and maintaining accurate records;
- develop your awareness of your interpersonal skills and consider how these could be enhanced;
- understand professional communication strategies when using email as a communication tool.

Introduction: the importance of communication

Whilst the whole of this book is dedicated to the development of knowledge and skills within a diverse preceptorship framework, it would be fair to say that all aspects of the framework have one single attribute in common; namely, they all rely on communication. The reason for this is quite straightforward. No doubt you will already be convinced of the fact that communication lies at the heart of nursing, so it will come as no surprise that communication and interpersonal skills also underpin all aspects of the preceptorship framework. Let's take some time to put this in context. Perhaps you could take the time now to review the index of this book. Everywhere you look, every theme of every chapter will somehow be tied up with some aspect of communication and/or interpersonal skills. For example, reflection and feedback would be impossible without communication, likewise teamwork, advocacy, conflict resolution; the list is endless.

We could go so far as to say that communication and interpersonal skills are at the heart of nursing, and are impossible to distance from care and compassion. The obvious conclusion here, of course, is that good communication and interpersonal skills equate to competent (caring) nursing. Your competence as a nurse will rely on your communication and interpersonal skills. Developing your professional practice will require ongoing development of these skills.

Communication and the NMC

The requirement for competent communication and interpersonal skills is clearly stated within the NMC's *The Code: Standards of Conduct, Performance and Ethics for Nurses and Midwives* (2008a). The four key standards for trustworthiness as a registrant include a requirement for the following:

- make the care of people your first concern, treating them as individuals and respecting their dignity;
- work with others to protect and promote the health and wellbeing of those in your care, their families and carers, and the wider community;
- provide a high standard of practice and care at all times;
- be open and honest, act with integrity and uphold the reputation of your profession (NMC, 2008a).

All of these four statements have communication implicitly at their core. Treating people as individuals will require appropriate communication, as will working with others, providing high standards of care and honesty. Yet the NMC does far more than just imply the need for communication and interpersonal skills: *The Code: Standards of Conduct, Performance and Ethics for Nurses and Midwives* (2008a) also outlines specific areas where professional standards in terms of communication must be upheld. We will look at record-keeping as one specific example further in the chapter. The key point to understand here is that throughout your nursing career your competence as a nurse will be grounded within your competence as a communicator. You can expect therefore that communication will be an ongoing theme throughout your preceptorship programme.

Interpersonal skills and communication

We already know that communication is important in nursing; for example, verbal communication (both spoken and written) is the primary way of transmitting vital information about patient issues (Racia, 2009). In addition, it is only through good communication and the development of the therapeutic relationship that nurses can identify the unique needs of patients (Foy and Timmins, 2004). Yet while we generally accept that communication is important in nursing, the fact is that we are not all naturally gifted in communication skills. While some people find communication relatively straightforward, others really struggle with this skill. Research suggests that communication and interpersonal skills are important to patients so that they:

- feel listened to;
- feel that their concerns are validated and not trivialised;
- feel supported;
- feel understood (Gilbert and Leahy, 2007).

The good news is that communication skills can be learnt and developed. To be a good communicator, however, you will need some self-awareness of your communication abilities to develop the required skills. In Chapters 2, 3 and 4 we looked extensively at issues related to developing skills in self-awareness and reflection, and how to set personal learning goals. It may be that after reading through these chapters you identified a number of areas related to your communication and/or interpersonal skills that require development. If so, then this chapter will be a significant aid to developing those skills.

Verbal communication

Considering that most of us use verbal communication daily and have done so since a very early age it is surprising that we do not all excel at this skill. In fact, it is widely accepted that despite the frequency of verbal communication, miscommunication of patient information occurs and has been identified as a major cause of health errors (Benjamin, 2001). While there are many facets to verbal miscommunication, some of the more common errors are related to overuse of jargon and specialist language (Foy and Timmins, 2004).

Case study: Jennifer explains an error of communication

I have been a registered nurse for over 30 years and I would have said that my communication skills were excellent; however, I recently had a reminder that it is just so easy to make a mistake through simple miscommunication. Last week I needed to attend a meeting and asked my manager what time it was and the venue. He told me it was at ten to 12 in seminar room 2. At 11.50 I turned up at seminar room 2 and found that the meeting was almost over. I couldn't believe what had happened. Instead of hearing that the meeting was from 10 a.m. to 12 noon, I heard this as ten minutes to 12 noon. It was a classic example of him saying one thing and me hearing something totally different. It made me realise just how easy it is to be complacent in communication, especially if you know people well and work with them often. It's just too easy to assume you know what is being said rather than make sure you have understood what is

continued opposite...

---

continued...

being said. On this occasion all that happened as a result of miscommunication was a missed meeting, but what if this was a time for medication administration, or the time an interpreter had been booked, or some other aspect of patient care? While we intended no harm, a patient really could have suffered because of our poor communication with each other. If I had one piece of advice to give to a newly registered nurse it would be never to let your standards of communication drop, don't ever assume that you have understood because mistakes can happen so easily. It takes two seconds to double check something and that is time worth spending if it prevents patients being harmed.

As a newly qualified nurse the risk of verbal miscommunication has particular significance for you. Firstly, you will be adjusting to a new practice environment, perhaps where the language and terminology is new or unfamiliar. Even if the language is familiar you will be using the language under different circumstances to what you may have previously been accustomed. Also, at this stage of your professional development you are more likely to experience a lack of communication confidence, perhaps even an unwillingness to communicate assertively when confronted with people who are rude or unco-operative (Bandura, 1977). The net effect of these situations will mean that if your verbal communication skills are met with a negative response you may well lose confidence and this in turn may lead to stress, anxiety and loss of confidence in your communication skills (Pajares, 2002). You may even avoid verbal communication altogether as a means to manage potential threats to your esteem (Racia, 2009). In Chapter 10 we will explore this situation even further in the context of nursing advocacy. For the time being we will focus on eliminating miscommunication by using a thoughtful and evidence-based approach to developing your verbal communication skills.

Active listening

The best way to improve your verbal communication skills is to develop your listening skills. Specifically, this will involve developing your active listening skills. Remember that you don't speak in order to hear your own voice: the reason you speak is to pass on information to others. If the information that you pass on is not clear then miscommunication will result. The only way you can check that your information has been clearly delivered is through using active listening strategies to check that your message has been conveyed clearly. Hearing is just one part of active listening; the majority of active listening involves recognition of non-verbal communication that often gets referred to as body language (McCabe and Timmins, 2006).

Activity 9.1: Communication

Active listening

This activity allows you to very quickly ascertain if active listening takes place amongst colleagues in your practice area. Without telling anyone what you are doing, try to observe a situation where verbal communication is being used. You may choose a meeting, handover or case conference for this exercise. Try to observe the following:

- When one person is talking, what are the other members of the group doing?
- What body language can you observe (facial expressions, fidgeting, body posture etc.)?

continued overleaf...

continued...

- How is information clarified? Are questions asked?
- What verbal or non-verbal signs are used that would indicate that information has been understood?
- Are there any verbal or non-verbal signs within the group that information has not been understood?
- What does the person communicating do to ensure that information has been understood?

As this activity is based on your own reflection, there is no outline answer at the end of the chapter.

Active listening should be employed equally in interactions between patients and colleagues as all that is required is to give the other person your full attention. It is not a passive behaviour; it involves prompts and phrases to encourage the other person to provide more explanation and to reflect on what is being said (Foy and Timmins, 2004). Active listening means that you are paying attention to *what* is being said and *how* it is being said. If you have not been understood or your message has been misinterpreted then listening to feedback will clarify this (Bach and Grant, 2009). Body postures and gestures such as head-nodding and facial expressions are prime ways to determine if your communication is clear and you are being understood (Foy and Timmins, 2004). Think back to Activity 9.1. Did you notice non-verbal active listening techniques within the group such as eye contact, head-nodding or facial expressions appropriate to what was being said? If you did not witness any of these it is quite likely that not everyone on the room was paying attention to what was being said. For this reason Bach and Grant (2009) argue that nurses should ask for confirmation or explanation if it is uncertain whether communication is understood.

Gibbons (1993) also suggests that one of the reasons that nurses do not actively listen is that their work is so action-orientated that they find it hard to be silent in their minds. This means that listening in the healthcare setting will require a deliberate commitment to fully engage with everyone, colleagues and staff alike (Foy and Timmins, 2004). There are many ways to ensure that this occurs. Active listening will therefore involve the following:

- looking directly at people when you are speaking and they are speaking to you;
- allowing someone to speak without interrupting, taking note of what they say and the body language they are using;
- making sure you reflect their feelings in your body language and your facial expression;
- observing the other person for feedback on your communication (McCabe and Timmins, 2006).

Research summary: the SBAR tool

In 2008 the NHS Institute for Innovation and Improvement endorsed the SBAR as an easy-to-remember tool consisting of standardised prompt questions that can be used to communicate patient information amongst health professionals. The tool was developed to allow staff to communicate assertively and effectively, reducing the need for repetition.

The four sections of SBAR include **S**ituation, **B**ackground, **A**ssessment and **R**ecommendation. Within each of the four categories, health professionals can use the

continued opposite...

continued...

tool to ensure information is passed on in a logical format and important detail is not lost. It is a particularly useful aid for inexperienced staff who may feel uncomfortable about giving a recommendation or communicating to senior staff. When each of the categories of SBAR is used sequentially the element of hinting and hoping can be eliminated. The SBAR tool is an ideal way to structure a telephone conversation to another health professional regarding a specific patient. An example of a staff nurse in a recovery unit ringing an on-call anaesthetist is provided as follows.

Situation – Identifying who you are and what unit you are calling from, the issue you are calling about and your concern(s)

Hi, this is Jodi Foster, staff nurse in the recovery unit. I'm calling about Mrs Valarie Bloomer, who has just arrived in the unit following an umbilical hernia repair. The reason for my call is I'm concerned about her pain.

Background – Identifying the patient with a short background history

Valarie Bloomer was given 10mg of morphine in theatre; however, she has not got any post-operative analgesia prescribed.

Assessment – Your concerns related to assessment (vital signs, increasing pain, etc.)

She is obviously in quite a lot of pain here with us. She is tachycardic and hypertensive, and she is verbally distressed; calling out in pain and unable to keep still in bed.

Recommendation – A suggestion as to a course of action including a time frame; for example, a change of medication dosage required immediately

Could you please return to the recovery room and review her analgesia? She is an ideal candidate for IV morphine boluses, a PCA for the ward and PRN paracetamol. Are you able to come now and prescribe this for her? (NHS (2008) Institute for Innovation and Improvement).

Written communication

As a nursing student you will have been provided with many opportunities to learn under the guidance and supervision of a mentor (Bach and Grant, 2009). However, for legal and ethical reasons some of the experiences that you undertook will have required constant overview and supervision by a mentor or registered nurse. One such example of this will have been documentation in patients' notes, records, charts, care plans, etc. While you may have had many opportunities to practise verbal communication skills independently, you will not have had the same opportunities for independent practice in record-keeping. In fact, the majority of the records you maintained as a student nurse will have been reviewed and countersigned by a qualified nurse.

This has of course all changed, and as a registered nurse you are now fully accountable for the records that you maintain. In law, what you write and record are viewed as part of your professional accountability and responsibility. In terms of culture shock, this is perhaps one of the biggest leaps you will need to make. Your literacy will no longer be judged or assessed through essays; it will now be judged in terms of your ability to deliver high quality care (Learner, 2006) and evidenced by concrete skills such as charting ability (Anders et al., 1995).

Standards for record-keeping

The NMC provides very clear guidelines and advice on the records you must keep as a nurse. The NMC *Record Keeping: Guidance for Nurses and Midwives* (2010b) provides clear advice for registrants on all aspects of record-keeping. This includes:

- key principles;
- confidentiality;
- access;
- disclosure;
- information systems;
- personal and professional knowledge and skills (NMC, 2010b).

Activity 9.2: Critical thinking

NMC Guidance for Record Keeping

Take the time now to access and read the current guidance on record-keeping for registrants. It is available on the NMC website and can be easily accessed at: **www.nmc-uk.org/Documents/Guidance/nmcGuidanceRecordKeepingGuidancefor NursesandMidwives.pdf**

Use this guidance to reflect on your own abilities as a record-keeper. To gain the most from this exercise you might like to use a recent sample of patient records that you have documented to assess yourself against the key areas within the guidance. Then use the results of your self-assessment to develop some clear goals for your professional development in your written record-keeping.

As this activity is based on your own reflection, there is no outline answer at the end of the chapter.

In addition, the professional expectations are clearly outlined by the NMC within *The Code: Standards of Conduct, Performance and Ethics for Nurses and Midwives* (2008a). In summary, these include the following.

- You must keep clear and accurate records of the discussions you have, the assessments you make, the treatment and medicines you give and how effective these have been.
- You must complete records as soon as possible after an event has occurred.
- You must not tamper with original records in any way.
- You must ensure that any entries you make in someone's paper records are clearly and legibly signed, dated and timed.

- You must ensure that any entries you make in someone's electronic records are clearly attributable to you.
- You must ensure that all records are kept securely (NMC, 2008a).

It may come as somewhat of a shock to realise the extent of your role and responsibility as a registrant in maintaining records of your care. Keep in mind also that the NMC frequently reviews and updates its guidance. The next update of guidance for record-keeping will take place in 2012. It will be a crucial part of your professional role that you investigate any changes to NMC guidance and make adjustments to your practice as required.

Record-keeping within information systems

One of the greatest challenges you will find as a registrant will be in maintaining your professional competence in a climate where the requirements for professional competence are in a constant state of change. Over recent years the need to adjust competence in record-keeping to meet the requirements of information systems has provided just one example of this. While email has made communication easier in terms of time, cost efficiency and geographical location (Hughes and Pakieser, 1999), it has also meant that nurses must develop skills in communicating competently via email. If you do use electronic communication with patients or colleagues you will need to be aware that you will be missing out on some of the key attributes of good interpersonal communication; namely, eye contact, body language and facial expression (Cleary and Freeman, 2005). If the interpersonal element is going to be an important aspect of ensuring clear communication you may need to review your communication method, perhaps using a Skype conversation with webcam, a video conference call or arranging a face-to-face meeting. In some cases indiscriminate use of email could be a source of stress or conflict (Cleary and Freeman, 2005). Remember that just because a communication method is available it is still your responsibility as a healthcare professional to ensure that the best communication method is being used.

Chapter summary

The purpose of this chapter was to look at the relationship between interpersonal skills and communication strategies. Throughout your professional career you will be required to identify appropriate communication strategies in order to deliver safe and effective care. To achieve this, you will need to self-assess and reflect on your interpersonal skills and consider how these could be enhanced to develop your communication skills.
In addition, you will need to be aware of current NMC guidance in relation to your written/verbal communication and maintaining accurate records. As developments in information systems are incorporated into nursing practice you will need to adapt and alter your communication strategies to ensure professional standards are not compromised.

Further reading

Bach, S and Grant, A (2009) *Communication and Interpersonal Skills for Nurses*. Exeter: Learning Matters.
This very easy-to-read book tackles implications of health policy, issues of culture and diversity and communication methods.

Ellis, R, Gates, B and Kenworthy, N (2003) *Interpersonal Communication in Nursing*, 2nd edn. London: Churchill Livingstone.
This is a useful book for understanding the theoretical concepts of communication into the analysis of everyday nursing situations. As well as being interesting to read, this book has the added benefit of encouraging reflective practice.

Useful websites

Electronic record-keeping is going to be implemented across the whole NHS to enhance communications across organisations and multidisciplinary teams. The activity, 'Electronic record keeping', provides a very good introduction to future development. You can find this on the Flying Start England website at:
www.flyingstartengland.nhs.uk/documentation

If you like to review the communication skills first visited as a student nurse you may find the 'Reviewing your communication skills' activity on the Flying Start NHS website. You can find this activity at: **www.flyingstart.scot.nhs.uk/learning-programmes/communication/interpersonal-skills.aspx**

Chapter 10
Advocacy

Preceptorship Framework and KSF

This chapter maps to the following elements of the Department of Health
Preceptorship Framework and the NHS Knowledge and Skills Framework.

Preceptorship Framework

- Advocacy
- Interpersonal skills
- Negotiation and conflict resolution
- Team-working
- Implement the Code and professional values

NHS Knowledge and Skills Framework

- Communication
- Personal and people development
- Quality
- Equality and diversity

Chapter aims

The aim of this chapter is to gain further understanding of the nurse's role as an advocate,
including professional implications for advocacy in practice. At the end of this chapter
you will be able to:

- identify your advocacy role as a member of the multidisciplinary team;
- recognise the attributes of assertiveness as opposed to aggression;
- understand the implications of advocacy in relation to the NMC code of conduct.

Introduction: the nurse as advocate

In the previous chapter we looked extensively at the links between interpersonal skills and
communication within a nursing context. We established that in order to deliver competent care
a registered nurse must be an excellent communicator, equally competent in written and verbal
communication. In particular, we discussed the need to maintain and develop competence in
interpersonal skills such as active listening in order to promote the therapeutic relationship and
thereby identify the unique needs of patients (Foy and Timmins, 2004). Throughout this chapter
we will be once again talking about communication and interpersonal skills, with a focus on
advocacy as a core dimension of communication.

Hanks (2010) suggests that advocacy for a patient is such an important aspect of current professional nursing care that it is considered to be a fundamental value of professional nursing. As a newly qualified nurse you will be expected to enact the role of patient advocate, using your interpersonal and communication skills to facilitate this aspect of your professional responsibility.

What is advocacy?

While most people would agree that advocacy is central to nursing care it is difficult to obtain a clear definition of the term (Zomorodi and Foley, 2009). The nursing literature classifies advocacy in three main ways:

- advocacy motivated by a patient's right to information and self-determination;
- advocacy as a right to personal safety;
- advocacy as a philosophical principle in nursing (Vaarito and Leino-Kilpi, 2005).

What most definitions of advocacy have in common is the focus of the nurse completing the desired wishes or needs of the patient (Zomorodi and Foley, 2009). Based on these definitions, it is not difficult to see why advocacy has been viewed for many years as the basis of the nurse–patient relationship (Curtin, 1979).

Being an advocate

Every time you undertake an aspect of nursing care you are in fact advocating for your patient. According to Zomorodi and Foley (2009), nurses express advocacy by creating an environment that is open and supportive to decision-making, using a knowledge of the person as an individual to define the relationship (Mallik, 1997). In other words, every time you involve your patient in a decision about their care you are expressing a form of advocacy. Of course, none of this would be possible without the required interpersonal and communication skills that we discussed in Chapter 9.

Activity 10.1: Leadership and management

Advocacy in practice

Take some time to reflect on a recent care event, perhaps the last shift you undertook. Can you think of examples of when you may have been a patient advocate? In particular, think of those situations where you discussed a particular patient need or personal choices. Some examples are provided below to get you started:

- a meal choice or particular dietary need;
- a decision regarding the time for physiotherapy, an outpatient appointment, a dressing change, a shower;
- a discussion on alternative medication options for analgesia;
- a plan for a home visit;
- a discussion about care package options;
- a choice of alternatives for group therapy.

continued opposite...

continued... •

Write down some personal examples and make some brief notes about the consequence of the advocacy event. In particular, pay attention to whether another member of the multidisciplinary team was involved during or as a consequence of the advocacy event.

As this activity is based on your own reflection, there is no outline answer at the end of the chapter.

Advocacy and the multidisciplinary team

Now that you have completed Activity 10.1, it should be very clear that acting as a nurse advocate very rarely means that you will be acting alone or in isolation. While advocacy is central to nursing (Hanks, 2010), advocacy will involve other members of the multidisciplinary team. In fact, some of the more common examples of advocacy cited by nurses include intervening on behalf of patients, speaking up and standing up for patients (Foley et al., 2000). Of course the implication here is that advocacy will require that communication and interpersonal skills are used in order to intervene, stand up and speak up, often to senior or more experienced people within the multidisciplinary team.

Case study: Grace reflects on being a patient advocate

I remember very early on after qualifying: I was on a night shift and one of my patients needed a chest x-ray. He was 83 years old, recovering from an operation and just exhausted. It was about 3 a.m. and his doctor wanted an x-ray but I really didn't want him going down a draughty corridor to the x-ray department and being pushed and pulled about. He was really upset as well; he obviously didn't want to go but it was a junior doctor and I just think she wanted the x-ray done and wasn't really thinking about what it would be like for the patient. In the end I put my foot down and insisted on a mobile x-ray on the ward. I had to argue a bit because the doctor didn't want hassle from the x-ray technician but in the end I got a mobile x-ray. It might seem a really small thing but for me it was the first time I really had to stand up for my patient as a newly qualified nurse. I was shaking with nerves but I also knew that if I didn't fight for my patient then no one else would do it and I just wasn't going to let this poor man be dragged around. I remember thinking, 'You're a nurse now, this is what nurses do'. Somehow that gave me courage so I just went for it.

As you are at a very early stage in your nursing career the communication and interpersonal skills required for patient advocacy may be one aspect of the nursing role that creates the most anxiety and seems the most daunting. You will be adjusting to a new practice environment, and using language or terminology under different circumstances to what you may have previously been accustomed as a student nurse. It is not uncommon for newly registered nurses to experience a lack of communication confidence, and you may find it very difficult to communicate assertively when confronted with people who are rude or unco-operative (Bandura, 1977). In the above case study, Grace had the confidence to speak up because she realised that she was the only person in a position to do so. She had to be assertive because there was no one else to fulfil this role. It should be clear, therefore, that the nature of advocacy will mean that you need to use assertive communication every day.

Advocate with confidence

In order to be an effective patient advocate you will need to have confidence in your own communication skills. If you lack confidence in your verbal communication skills and are met with a negative response, you may well lose confidence altogether, leading to stress and anxiety (Pajares, 2002). You may even avoid verbal communication altogether as a means to manage potential threats to your esteem (Racia, 2009). If you find yourself avoiding verbal communication, you will be failing as a patient advocate. In order to be an effective patient advocate you will need to have confidence in your own ability to communicate, and to communicate assertively.

Assertive communication

Assertive communication has been defined as the ability to express your thoughts, ideas and feelings without undue anxiety or exposure to others (Balzer-Riley, 2000). Assertiveness is a skill in itself and like all skills needs to be learnt and developed (Bach and Grant, 2009). While most nurses may recognise that to be a patient advocate they will need to be an assertive communicator, some nurses do not communicate assertively because they worry what others may think of them; that anxiety is grounded in a lack of confidence (Poroch and McIntosh, 1995). As a newly qualified nurse these particular concerns may be very real to you. Assertive communication plays a very big role in terms of negotiation and conflict resolution that we will discuss in Chapter 11. However, for the time being we will focus on the skills required to use assertive communication within the multidisciplinary team in order to fulfil your role as a patient advocate.

> ### Research summary: key features of assertive behaviour
>
> While assertive communication and behaviour have many different attributes the following list outlines some of the core features of assertiveness:
> - being open and honest (with yourself and others);
> - listening to other people's points of view;
> - showing an understanding of others situations;
> - expressing your own ideas clearly, honestly and with care;
> - standing up for yourself;
> - having self-respect and respect for other people;
> - being clear about your point and not being sidetracked (Willis and Daisley, 1995).

Assertive advocacy

It is generally accepted that nurses are in the best position to advocate (Llewellyn and Northway, 2010) and that communication is a fundamental feature of advocacy. In the INSA bulletin (2010) it is suggested that assertive advocacy involves two core communication strategies. These include:

- ensuring verbal communication matches non-verbal behaviours;
- sincerity in all comments with patients and members of the multidisciplinary team (INSA bulletin, 2010).

Another feature of assertive advocacy is through the development of a partnership approach to patient care. While patients may have less power and control in a healthcare setting, this does not mean that they are passive participants in their healthcare needs. In order for you to be an assertive patient advocate it is first important to establish the views and contributions by patients regarding their care preferences, rather than being in a one-way information-giving relationship (Jarrett and Payne, 1995). In this way nurses can use assertive communication to empower patients to question professionals' decisions and to become involved in the decision-making process (Markanday, 1997).

Assertiveness versus aggression

If a partnership approach to advocacy is not employed, this can create a situation where your communication is interpreted as aggression. If patients interpret your communication as aggressive they may feel dominated and this can lead to dependence (Foy and Timmins, 2004). Additionally, if you are aggressive in your advocacy you may inadvertently pass on more information than the patient is prepared to absorb (Foy and Timmins, 2004). This can be especially true for older patients who have been socialised into and are comfortable with a more passive role in relation to healthcare decision-making (Mitchell, 1997). In order to ensure that your communication is interpreted as assertive rather than aggressive you will need to have a good grasp of interpersonal skills including the ability to actively listen and interpret non-verbal communication, particularly body language (Foy and Timmins, 2004).

Case study: Claire speaks of her experience with an 'aggressive' nurse

When my mother was 73 she had minor surgery in a day care unit. The nurse was very keen for my mother to eat before she went home; however, my mum felt a little nauseated and didn't feel like eating the tuna sandwich on offer. The nurse adopted a really aggressive approach to this, stating that unless she ate we would have to stay. Rather than offering my mum some medication for nausea and then asking what she preferred to eat, she just launched into a long explanation on the cause of post-operative nausea. Rather than helpful advice and a discussion on alternatives, my poor mum was subjected to a totally unnecessary lecture. I remember throwing away the tuna sandwich and buying my mum something she actually fancied from the cafeteria. If I hadn't been there to sort all this out I'm not sure my mum would have got home that day.

It is important to realise also that there is a possibility of your assertive communication turning into aggressive behaviour when dealing with members of the multidisciplinary team. As a newly registered nurse it is easy to fall into the trap of thinking that you must 'prove' yourself in order to gain respect, and that being dominant is one way to achieve this. Unfortunately the only effect that this behaviour will have is to alienate people from you and to risk incurring an unwanted label.

Case study: Samuel discusses communication skills

A newly qualified nurse started in our clinic quite recently and she is having a very difficult time with her colleagues. It started during case meetings when she would interrupt during case reviews with her opinion of what needed to be done, or an observation about her own patients. The other nurses in the department

continued overleaf...

continued...

> *have tolerated this so far but during the last meeting I noticed she was being very aggressive in order to get her point across. We all realise she is just trying to establish herself in a new work environment, but she is going about getting respect in all the wrong ways. I just don't think she knows the difference between being assertive and being aggressive. It can't carry on like this so I'm going to do some reflections on our case meetings with her. It's obvious she is a confident communicator and that's great, but at the moment she is just going about it in the wrong way.*

When you are aggressive you are essentially using your personal anger to persuade another person (McCabe and Timmins, 2006). Aggression can be expressed through a variety of means, but the most common tend to be use of a loud voice, finger wagging or pointing, standing over people or invading personal space (McCabe and Timmins, 2006). It is a method of getting your own way and disregarding the consequences (Willis and Daisley, 1995). If you use this method to communicate with members of the multidisciplinary team the consequence will be a lack of respect; you will annoy others and be generally disliked (McCabe and Timmins, 2006). Most importantly, you will fail as a patient advocate and as a result their care will be compromised by your inappropriate communication.

Activity 10.2: Communication

Assertiveness in action

This activity is designed to allow you to explore how you might use assertive communication skills to resolve a problem related to patient care. Start by reading the short scenario and then take some time to think through a course of action you might take. Make some brief notes about how you would deal with this situation in an assertive manner.

Scenario

You arrive for your rostered Saturday shift to find that the senior nurse in charge has called in sick and the nurse in charge of the night shift tells you that a replacement has not been found. You are newly qualified and this is your first Saturday shift in this ward. The nurse handing over tells you that when she was newly qualified the same thing happened to her and she just had to 'get on with it'. She tells you that 'they will probably send someone from the bank'. You feel very overwhelmed by this situation; you do not feel that you are able to take charge of the shift given your level of knowledge and your inexperience.

How would you use assertive communication to deal with this situation?

There is a brief outline answer to this activity at the end of the chapter.

Advocacy and the NMC

It should come as no surprise that advocacy is one of the key features of *The Code: Standards of Conduct, Performance and Ethics for Nurses and Midwives* (NMC, 2008a). The professional requirement of a nurse outlines very clearly where your accountability and responsibility lie in relation to advocacy:

- You must act as an advocate for those in your care, helping them to access relevant health and social care, information and support.
- You must listen to the people in your care and respond to their concerns and preferences.
- You must support people in caring for themselves to improve and maintain their health.
- You must recognise and respect the contribution that people make to their own care and wellbeing (NMC, 2008a).

There is obviously a significant requirement for all registrants to be competent in the types of interpersonal and communication skills that will make advocacy possible. Remember also that as you progress throughout your career you will be required to develop your advocacy skills, and the needs of patients and clients. While your role and responsibility in relation to patient care may alter over time, the essence of nursing care promoting empowerment through advocacy will remain consistent (Foy and Timmins, 2004).

Chapter summary

Throughout this chapter we have discussed the role of the nurse as an advocate, including professional implications for advocacy in practice. In order to be a competent patient advocate you will need to utilise interpersonal and communication skills in order to understand the healthcare needs of your patients. You will use these same skills when employing your advocacy role as a member of the multidisciplinary team. We have also discussed that one of the key elements of competent advocacy is to recognise the attributes of assertiveness versus aggression and the implications of advocacy in relation to NMC accountability and responsibility. In the next chapter we will be exploring interpersonal skills, communication and advocacy once again, this time in the context of conflict resolution and managing difficult situations.

Activities: brief outline answer

Activity 10.2: Assertiveness in action (page 96)

This activity required you to think about using assertive communication to deal with a difficult practice situation. Obviously there are many ways of using assertive communication, and this outline answer merely suggests one example for resolution.

You could use assertive communication to speak with your colleague on the night shift, explaining that you would appreciate her help to resolve the situation. You could explain that given your current level of experience it would not be safe for her to leave the ward without a senior nurse as a replacement. You could ask some direct questions that gave you an idea of what had been done so far to find a replacement. This may involve enquiring about what site manager has been involved and if the site manager is aware that you are recently qualified. You could contact the site manager yourself and explain the situation, making it clear that a satisfactory replacement will ensure safe patient care. You could even suggest some alternative actions; for example, transferring a more experienced nurse from another area to your ward or asking for the site manager to lend assistance for aspects of care with which you are unfamiliar.

Further reading

Arnold, E and Boggs, K (2007) *Interpersonal Relationships: Professional Communication Skills for Nurses*, 5th edn. Philadelphia, PA: WB Saunders.

This book provides fundamental information about communication theory and applications for all nurses to develop specific aspects of the nurse–patient relationship.

Useful websites

www.businessballs.com/self-confidence-assertivness.htm

This is a very useful and practical website for developing further skills in assertive communication.

Flying Start England provides some useful links to websites that are useful resources on assertiveness for both yourself and patients in your care. You can find these links via the 'Assertiveness web search' activity at: **www.flyingstartengland.nhs.uk/communicationassertiveness**

Chapter 11
Negotiation and conflict resolution

Chapter aims

By the end of this chapter you will be able to:
- identify the difficult situations that may arise in the workplace;
- identify the common causes of conflict within the practice setting and appreciate the impact of conflict on people and the work environment;
- consider different strategies to manage conflict;
- identify the causes of patient complaints;
- identify steps that can be taken to reduce the likelihood of complaints;
- understand the steps that should be taken to respond to patient complaints.

Introduction

As a nurse you will come across many difficult situations during your career. These may arise because of problems with organisational structures or processes, at a macro level, or occur at a more personal level in your interactions with colleagues, patients, service users and carers. In some of these situations conflict may arise in others, and you may find yourself in a position where you are unsure how to respond. This may be because you lack the skills, knowledge or experience necessary, or because systems and processes are not in place that will support you to take appropriate actions. While avoiding a difficult situation can be very attractive, there are invariably consequences if you don't deal with them at the time and in some cases these could have serious repercussions for yourself or others involved. The aim of this chapter is to explore how conflict may arise within the nursing environment and how the skills of negotiation and conflict resolution can be used to prevent the negative consequences that occur where conflict is not resolved. This chapter also deals with patient complaints as areas of challenge, and explores how best to manage them.

Conflict

Conflict can be defined as *a process involving two or more people where one perceives the opposition of another* (Almost, 2006, page 447). The word 'conflict' tends to have a negative connotation, but an environment where conflict never occurs is not necessarily a good one either for the people who work there or for patients. This is because conflict is often necessary for changes to be made; in a conflict-free workplace the status quo is being maintained in order to 'keep everyone happy'. This status quo can be detrimental to those involved, who can become frustrated and angry, because their concerns are not being addressed, and also to the service they deliver if systems and processes are never challenged. A certain level of conflict therefore can be healthy if it is managed appropriately.

Causes of conflict

Conflict arises because there are differences between people's values, beliefs, needs, desires, responsibilities, assumptions or expectations. Almost (2006) groups the causes of conflict into these three areas:

- individual characteristics, e.g. value differences, demographic dissimilarity or generational diversity;
- interpersonal factors, e.g. lack of trust, injustice or disrespect, inadequate or poor communication;
- organisational factors, e.g. interdependence or changes due to restructuring.

Activity 11.1: Reflection

Your experience of conflict

Reflect on a situation where there was conflict in your workplace. Can you identify what the cause of conflict was? What was the outcome?

As this is a reflective activity, there is no outline answer at the end of this chapter.

Consequences of conflict

Almost (2006) grouped the consequences of conflict in nursing work under four headings:

1. individual effects, e.g. job stress or dissatisfaction, absenteeism, intent to leave, increased grievances, psychosomatic complaints, negative emotions;

2. interpersonal relationships (negative), e.g. negative perception of others, hostility, avoidance;
3. organisational effects, e.g. reduced coordination and collaboration, reduced productivity;
4. interpersonal relationships (positive), e.g. stronger relationships, team cohesiveness.

Any of the consequences under the first three headings can clearly impact negatively, not only on the individual but also on the quality of patient care. The focus of Almost's (2006) concept analysis is on nursing work environments and does not explore conflict where it involves service users and carers. Where conflict arises with service users or carers, the consequences may include some of those listed above, but if not managed appropriately the consequences may also include complaints or abuse, either verbal or physical, as we shall now see.

Violence in the NHS

Healthcare professionals as an occupational group are second only to the protective service professions (police, fire and prison officers) in experiencing violence at work (Packham, 2010). Following the publication of The National Audit Office's report, *A Safer Place to Work – protecting NHS hospital and ambulance staff from violence and aggression* (NAO, 2003), a number of recommendations were made, including a standardised approach to staff training on conflict resolution with a national syllabus to ensure consistency of training. All health bodies are now required to take into account the guidance provided by the NHS Security Management Service. Courses on conflict resolution must cover:

- verbal and non-verbal communication skills;
- recognising warning signs;
- cultural awareness;
- de-escalation techniques.

Separate guidance exists for staff working in mental health and learning disability services with learning outcomes specific to these areas, including restraint-related risks.

Following the implementation of the measures arising from the NAO (2003) report, the NHS Security Management Service commissioned a survey by Ipsos MORI in 2010 to measure the progress made (see research summary).

Research summary: violence against frontline NHS staff

An Ipsos MORI telephone survey of 2,202 frontline healthcare professionals looking at violence against frontline NHS staff found that:
- 32% of staff said that they have been verbally abused or verbally threatened by a patient in the last 12 months;
- 18% of staff said that they had been verbally abused or verbally threatened by a member of the public (not a patient);
- 5% of staff said that they had been physically assaulted by a patient;
- 1% of staff said that they have been assaulted by a member of the public (not a patient).

The staff groups most likely to experience violence are:

continued overleaf...

continued...

- nurses in accident and emergency departments;
- security staff;
- inpatient nurses;
- staff in complaint roles (e.g. PALs).

The main factors that contributed to any verbal or physical abuse from members of the public or patients are detailed in Table 11.1.

Consequence of the patient's mental health condition	19%
Person was under the influence of alcohol	19%
Length of time waiting to be seen by a health professional	18%
Problems understanding information and/or instructions	16%
Consequence of the patient's medical condition	10%
Dissatisfaction with service/treatment, etc.	9%
Concern about their condition	8%
Person was under the influence of recreational drugs	8%
Concern about another patient's condition	5%
The feeling that they should be prioritised over other patients	5%
Frustration/anger	4%
High/unreasonable expectations	4%

Table 11.1: Factors in abuse against frontline NHS staff
Source: Ipsos MORI (2010)

Staff who had attended conflict resolution training were found to be more aware of the NHS security policies and procedures. There was a significant minority of staff who accepted workplace abuse as part of their job and/or failed to report it and there is therefore a need to encourage better reporting as this can enhance outcomes for staff.

If you have not yet attended conflict resolution training, discuss with your manager what training is available to you at work that you can attend; it is usually part of mandatory training so regular sessions should be available to you.

Conflict management styles or the art of negotiation

The way people respond to conflict can have a direct impact on the level of conflict in the workplace. A number of different conflict management styles are described in the literature (Rahim, 2010). The Thomas–Kilmann Conflict Mode Instrument (TKI) (Thomas and Kilmann,

1974) describes five different styles for handling conflict, based on a person's assertiveness (need to satisfy own concerns) and their co-operativeness (need to satisfy others' concerns).

The five styles are shown in Figure 11.1.

Assertiveness ↑	**Competing**			**Collaborating**
		Compromising		
	Avoiding			**Accommodating**
	Co-operativeness →			

Figure 11.1: The Thomas–Kilmann conflict management styles (Thomas, 1992, see Acknowledgements)

Competing

The competing style is assertive but unco-operative. In a conflict situation you are out to win. It can be seen as aggressive or dominating. It is often used by managers, people higher up in the hierarchy and by those who believe that their knowledge and/or experience gives them the authority to state what is needed or what should be done. This approach is appropriate in an emergency.

Collaborating

This style is high on both assertiveness and co-operativeness, recognising the needs of all parties involved. With this approach all views are considered in order to reach a consensus but as a consequence this approach can take longer to achieve resolution so only appropriate where there is time to do this.

Compromising

The solution reached through compromise will only partially satisfy each person involved. It is usually used where the collaborative approach has been unsuccessful, as a temporary solution or where a consensus cannot be achieved.

Accommodating

This style is low on assertion and high on co-operation. The accommodator will 'give in' because they believe that the issue is more important to the other party, they are arguing from a weak standpoint or because they believe that there may be the opportunity for calling in a favour in the future.

Avoiding

This style is commonly used in nursing (Vivar, 2006) and often seen in the newly registered nurse where the conflict involves someone with greater authority. The avoider is low on assertion and co-operation and chooses to avoid the conflict completely.

Depending on the cause of conflict, a more facilitative negotiating style may be better adopted. Negotiation involves discussion aimed at reaching an agreement and therefore is applicable to the collaborating and compromising styles and is appropriate where more time is available. While some people may predominantly use one style, it is important to be able to develop skills in using all of the above styles and recognise which ones are best used in any given situation and which styles are inappropriate. You can explore this more in the next activity.

Activity 11.2: Decision-making

When not to use a conflict management style

Consider the five conflict management styles that have been described. Can you identify situations for each style where it would be inappropriate to use that approach?

There is a brief outline answer to this activity at the end of the chapter.

Case study: Jason's off-duty

Jason has been working in his new post for two months and has noticed that none of his off-duty requests have been given. He feels that this is unfair but hasn't said anything yet (avoidance) because he doesn't want to be seen as difficult but it is impacting on his family life. So when the next off-duty schedule comes out and he has not received any of his requests again, he decides to talk to Ahmet, the unit manager. Ahmet stops him part way through his request and informs him that he is the manager and he must ensure the unit is covered and that once the off-duty is out it cannot be changed (competitive). Jason then has to decide whether to back down (accommodate) or to explore a compromise by agreeing to accept the current off-duty but discuss with Ahmet how the off-duty can be managed more fairly for all staff in the future. He tells Ahmet that he understands that patients must come first when planning the off-duty and asks whether he can be involved in the development of the next off-duty so that he can better understand why decisions are made as to who works which shifts; Ahmet agrees, a compromise has been reached.

Skills for conflict resolution

The key skill required for conflict resolution is effective communication (see Chapters 9 and 10), in particular the skill of active listening. You also need to be able to recognise where conflict exists or has the potential to arise, if not managed appropriately. Early recognition can enable you to defuse the situation before it escalates.

The warning signs of conflict

Conflict can develop over time or occur with little warning. Where conflict is occurring between two or more people who are avoiding confronting the issues, the possible signs may be:

- increased sickness by one or more members of staff involved;
- avoidance of working with each other/taking different breaks;
- criticism of the staff member's actions or ideas to others.

Where conflict is more immediate and aggressive in nature, warning signs may include:

- negative body language (e.g. eye rolling, head shaking, crossing of arms);
- increase in voice volume;
- direct and prolonged eye contact;
- increased respiratory rate.

In cases like this it is important to respond quickly to the situation in order to defuse it. A model often taught as part of conflict resolution training is CUDSA (Davis, 2007).

A communication model for resolving conflict

CUDSA is a five-step model which can be useful as an aide memoire in how to respond to someone where conflict has arisen (Nelson-Jones, 2006):

Confront the problem/situation
Understand each other's position
Define the problem
Search for a solution
Agree

It does require both parties to engage in discussion as they try to understand the issue of concern from both perspectives and agree a solution. For example, consider a patient who is becoming increasingly angry because they are waiting to go home but their medication to take home has not arrived from the pharmacy. Recognising that there is an issue, the nurse talks to the patient and explains why there is a delay, because the doctor has only just completed the list of medications for the pharmacist. The patient explains that the person taking them home needs to be back by a certain time and cannot wait much longer. The problem is therefore the limited time the patient has. A possible solution may be that the friend collects the medication from the pharmacy and brings them to the ward so that the nurse can then finalise the patient's discharge.

Patient complaints

Patient complaints are a potential cause of conflict and are increasing in number as patients become more aware of their rights and their expectations increase. The NHS Constitution sets out a patient's rights with regard to complaints and the NHS's commitment to responding to them (see Table 11.2).

You (the patient) have the right:	The NHS also commits:
to have any complaint you make about NHS services dealt with efficiently and to have it properly investigated	to ensure you are treated with courtesy and you receive appropriate support throughout the handling of a complaint; and the fact that you have complained will not adversely affect your future treatment (pledge)

continued overleaf...

continued...

to know the outcome of any investigation into your complaint	when mistakes happen, to acknowledge them, apologise, explain what went wrong and put things right quickly and effectively (pledge)
to take your complaint to the independent Health Service Ombudsman, if you are not satisfied with the way your complaint has been dealt with by the NHS	to ensure that the organisation learns lessons from complaints and claims and uses these to improve NHS services (pledge)
to make a claim for judicial review if you think you have been directly affected by an unlawful act or decision of an NHS body	
to compensation where you have been harmed by negligent treatment	

Table 11.2: The NHS Constitution (NHS, 2010b)

Since April 2009 the NHS has adopted a simpler, two-stage process for managing patient complaints. Step one (local resolution) is for the patient to raise the matter in writing or by speaking directly to the practitioner or their organisation. Step two is taken where the patient is unhappy with the outcome and can refer the matter to the Parliamentary and Health Services Ombudsman. The aim of the new approach is to move from a process-focused approach to an outcome approach whereby a patient-centred 'complaints plan' is developed that enables a collaborative partnership between the complainant and the complaints manager that looks at the steps that need to be taken to improve services (Holmes-Bonney, 2010). It is important that you are fully aware of the procedures for handling a complaint in your organisation. If you have not received training on this yet in your organisation, or need a refresher, you should undertake Activity 11.3.

Activity 11.3: Evidence-based practice and research

Local policy on patient complaints

Find a copy of your organisation's complaints policy and read through it.

Check your organisation's website for information for patients on making a complaint.

Arrange to meet with your local Patient Advice and Liaison Service (PALS) to discuss their role and how they can also support and advise you.

Look at the PALS website: **www.pals.nhs.uk/**

As this is an activity for you to develop your knowledge, there is no outline answer at the end of this chapter.

Causes of patient complaints

Two recent reports give an indication of the common causes of complaints. The Patient Opinion website **www.patientopinion.org.uk/** report, *In their words. What patients think about our NHS* (Patient Opinion, 2011), identifies the key issues that patients have with NHS healthcare services. The Parliamentary Health Ombudsman's report published in 2010 reviewed the complaints referred to it between 2009 and 2010 by patients who had been unhappy with the way that the complaint had been handled locally (see Table 11.3).

Patient opinion report	Ombudsman's report
Staff attitudes (33%)	Clinical care and treatment (36%)
Care and compassion (29%)	Attitudes of staff (10%)
Poor or miscommunication between patient and service (25%)	Diagnosis: delay, failure to diagnose, misdiagnosis (9%)
Lack of responsiveness by staff (22%)	Communication and information (including confidentiality) (8%)

Table 11.3: Causes of patients' complaints

The Ombudsman's report also identifies the reasons why patients had referred their complaints to them, having been unsatisfied with the response at a local level. These were identified as:

*   poor explanation;
*   response incomplete;
*   unnecessary delay;
*   factual errors in response to complaints;
*   no acknowledgement of mistake;
*   failure to understand the complaint and outcome sought by complainant;
*   communication with complainant unhelpful, ineffective, disrespectful.

As you can see, poor communication crops up both as a cause of the initial complaint but also in how it is handled. In many cases responding appropriately at the time of the initial complaint can prevent the matter from escalating further.

Responding to a patient's complaint

If a patient makes a complaint to you it is important that you do not dismiss it but listen very carefully to what they are saying:

*   Face the person and give them your full attention.
*   Listen actively to what they are saying; observe their body language (is it congruent with what they are saying, is there more that they are not saying?).
*   When they have finished speaking, paraphrase what you understand they have said.

- Check that you are correct and agree what the issues are; try to avoid blame and focus on solutions.
- Agree a course of action and be clear as to what outcomes the patient is expecting.

When a patient makes a complaint it is easy to feel defensive, but listening to their concerns and responding to them may resolve the issue on the spot. If this is not possible then seek further guidance from a colleague or talk to your PALS representative if one is available to you as they have considerable experience in managing patient complaints.

Chapter summary

This chapter has explored the concepts of conflict and conflict resolution and the management of patient complaints which, when poorly handled, can also lead to conflict. Central to these areas is the use of effective communication skills, which can be used to pick up cues and used to defuse potentially escalating problems.

Activities: brief outline answer

Activity 11.2: When not to use a conflict management style (page 104)

Examples of situations where it would be inappropriate for you to use specific conflict management style have been suggested by Rahim (2010) as:

- accommodating – where you know the other party is wrong or decision being made is unethical or the issue is important to you;
- avoiding – where an issue is important to yourself or you are responsible for the decision, the issue must be resolved quickly;
- competing – where the issue is not really important to you, for complex decisions where collaboration is important;
- collaborating – where a quick decision is required;
- compromising – where one party is more dominant.

Further reading

Fisher, R and Ury, W (2003) *Getting to Yes: Negotiating an Agreement Without Giving In*, 2nd edn. London: Random House Group.
A good introduction to the art of negotiation.

Harris, T (1995) *I'm OK – You're OK.* London: Arrow Books.
Although quite old now this is a quick and easy introduction to transactional analysis and can be helpful in understanding interrelationships.

Useful websites

There are some useful links to web resources on the Flying Start NHS website which will provide you with further guidance on conflict resolution. You will find these at: **www.flyingstart.scot.nhs.uk/ learning-programmes/communication/conflict-resolution.aspx**

There is a set of scenarios on the Flying Start England website which you will find useful to work through to test your conflict resolution skills. They can be found at: **www.flyingstartengland.nhs. uk/conflictresolution**

The NHS Business Services Authority website has a section on security management with a range of information and resources available including information regarding conflict resolution training: **www.nhsbsa.nhs.uk/Index.aspx**

Chapter 12
Implementing the Code and professional values

Preceptorship Framework and KSF

This chapter maps to the following elements of the Department of Health Preceptorship Framework and the NHS Knowledge and Skills Framework.

Preceptorship Framework
- Implementing the Code and professional values
- Increasing knowledge and clinical skills
- Understanding policies and procedures
- Confidence in applying evidence-based practice

NHS Knowledge and Skills Framework
- Communication
- Personal and people development
- Health, safety and security
- Quality

Chapter aims

The aim of this chapter is to explore professionalism and accountability. By the end of this chapter you will be able to:

- reflect on implications for you in becoming a registered nurse;
- appreciate the importance of demonstrating professional behaviour;
- reflect on your professional values;
- explain the difference between responsibility and accountability;
- explain the different types of accountability and their relevance to yourself.

Introduction

During your pre-registration nursing programme the course will have addressed the concepts of professionalism and accountability and it is highly likely that there were learning outcomes that you had to achieve in practice that included your ability to demonstrate professional behaviour. Accountability, however, was probably just a theoretical concept which did not become real until your first day as a registered nurse. As a student you will have had protected status because the registered nurses you worked with will have been accountable for your actions, but at the moment of registration you became both responsible and accountable for your actions. The implications of being responsible and accountable for one's own actions are one of the key areas that cause concern for the newly registered nurse (Higgens et al., 2010) and so this chapter aims to clarify for you how your role has changed as you have moved from student to registered nurse in relation to becoming a professional and the accountability that comes with it.

Becoming a professional

As a student you will have been expected to demonstrate professional behaviour throughout your programme. As a registered nurse this expectation will continue but takes on greater significance as not only do you now hold accountability for your actions but you will also be seen as a role model by healthcare students and colleagues who will look to you for guidance on what being a professional means. The way you practise as a professional will be strongly influenced by your values and it is quite likely that these have changed as you have progressed through your programme leading to registration. This is part of professional socialisation, whereby you have learnt what it means to be a nurse by observing the behaviour of other nurses (Leners et al., 2005).

What does it mean to be a professional?

There is no real consensus on the characteristics of a profession (Chitty, 2005); but common themes are:

- a defined body of knowledge;
- altruistic service to society;
- a code of ethics;
- accountability;
- autonomy;
- regulation of the profession following completion of an educational programme;
- existence of a professional body (Chitty, 2005; Cooke and Philpin, 2008; Hall and Ritchie, 2009).

The Royal College of Nursing, in its paper, *Defining Nursing* (RCN, 2004), differentiates between nursing and professional nursing by saying:

> *The distinction does not lie in the type of task performed nor in the level of skill that is required to perform a particular task. As for all professional practice, the difference lies in:*
>
> - *the clinical judgement inherent in the processes of assessment, diagnosis, prescription, and evaluation;*
> - *the knowledge that is the basis of the assessment of need and the determination of action to meet the need;*
> - *the personal accountability for all decisions and actions, including the decision to delegate to others;*
> - *the structured relationship between the nurse and the patient which incorporates professional regulation and a code of ethics within a statutory framework.*

The definition by the RCN incorporates many of the characteristics listed above but gives a greater insight into the expectation by others of you as a professional nurse and some of the values and behaviours you should be demonstrating.

Activity 12.1: Reflection

What does professional behaviour look like?

What behaviour was expected of you as a student that demonstrated professionalism?

There is a brief outline answer to this activity at the end of the chapter.

Unsurprisingly, the behaviours expected of you as a student will be the same as those expected of you as a registered nurse; the crucial change is that the NMC's Code (2008a) now also applies to you in its full extent as you are now fully accountable for your actions in upholding the Code.

It is likely that you will be very familiar with the Code (NMC, 2008a) but it is worth taking time to read it again with the knowledge that this is no longer something to which you are aspiring but something that you are required to follow at all times.

Professional values

The values you hold will have been developed over a number of years and will have been influenced by many factors including your family and friends, your educational experiences, your culture and any religious beliefs you may have. These values will influence your own attitudes and beliefs about nursing and so indirectly impact on your professional behaviour.

Activity 12.2: Reflection

Developing professional values

Think back on the reasons why you became a nurse. At your interview or in your application you may have discussed what was important to you and what you believed nursing to be. Have these ideals and values changed? If so, what may have led to any changes?

As this is a reflective activity, there is no outline answer at the end of this chapter.

During your pre-registration nursing programme you will probably have explored professional values in the classroom and these will have been further developed and refined as you were socialised into the world of nursing (Maben et al., 2007). Bandura and MacDonald (1963) found role models to be the most influential in developing or changing values and it is likely that you can recall key people you came into contact with during your programme who had a significant impact on you and influenced the way you enact your role as a nurse. One of the greatest challenges for newly registered nurses is when they find that organisational constraints mean that they have to compromise their professional values. This is discussed further in the research summary.

Research summary: constraints on professional values

In a longitudinal study, Maben et al. (2007) examined the experience of newly qualified nurses in implementing their ideals and values in today's health service. Three cohorts of students (*n=72*) completed a questionnaire during the last week of their programme and were asked to describe their ideals and values for practice as a qualified nurse. The responses were divided into three domains:

- embracing the delivery of patient-centred holistic care;
- the delivery of high quality care;
- care influenced by a theoretical knowledge base and research evidence.

An in-depth interview was undertaken with 26 of the original students at 4–6 months and 11–15 months post-qualification, and a further questionnaire sent to them three years after qualification. The research found that once qualified their ability to implement their espoused values and ideals was hampered by both professional and organisational constraints, in particular high workloads and high patient turnover. They also reported a change in the range of activities they now undertook, with a move from a patient-focused role giving direct and patient-orientated care to a more managerial, co-ordinating role which lessened their ability further to practise in a way that was congruent with their ideals and values. As a consequence the majority of the nurses felt they had to compromise their ideals, with a third feeling crushed and finding the only way to cope was to lower their expectations.

The failure by nurses to uphold their professional values is encapsulated in a recent report of the Health Service Ombudsman (Parliamentary and Health Service Ombudsman, 2011), which found major failings in the care of older patients, particularly with regard to the attitudes of healthcare staff to patients, a lack of respect for individuality and a lack of sensitivity, compassion and professionalism – all core professional values. The findings in the report are unfortunately not unique; local and national patient surveys and websites where patients provide feedback on their experiences of our healthcare system also identify major concerns regarding staff attitudes and the lack of care and compassion patients receive (Patient Opinion, 2011) and demonstrate vividly the impact that a failure to uphold your professional values can have on patients and their carers.

At times you may find your personal values also come into conflict with your professional values or even with those of a patient you are caring for. For example, you may believe in the sanctity of life and that as a nurse you should always seek to improve the health of your patients. However, if a patient's religious beliefs or personal values lead them to refuse certain care interventions such as a blood transfusion or a medical or therapeutic intervention this may cause an internal conflict for you as you try to reconcile your values and beliefs with the professional value of respecting a patient's wishes.

Professional values are encapsulated within the NMC's Code (NMC, 2008a), which has four key statements each, which are then explored in more depth. The key statements encapsulating our professional values are:

- *make the care of people your first concern, treating them as individuals and respecting their dignity;*
- *work with others to protect and promote the health and wellbeing of those in your care, their families and carers, and the wider community;*
- *provide a high standard of practice and care at all times;*
- *be open and honest, act with integrity and uphold the reputation of your profession* (NMC, 2008a, page 2).

Remember that at all times you are personally accountable for your actions and omissions and that failing to demonstrate these values through your practice could result in you being required to justify your decision not to uphold them.

Accountability

Accountability is at the very centre of professional practice. As discussed earlier, it is an important characteristic of a profession but more importantly it ensures that the public can have trust in the care you deliver.

There is no one definition of accountability, but put at its simplest, accountability is about being answerable for your actions ('being called to account') and is often related to, and sometimes muddled with, responsibility. The difference between the two is that responsibility relates to your acceptance of a duty that is within your sphere of competence and the carrying out of that duty, but accountability requires you to be answerable for the actions you undertake in fulfilling that duty. As a registered nurse you are answerable not only for your actions but also for any omissions. This means that at all times you must be able to justify any decisions you make which result in a specific course of action or inaction (NMC, 2009c).

A framework for accountability

Most nurses are very clear that they are answerable to the NMC for their actions. However, it is not always appreciated that you can also be held to account for your actions to the public and your patients through criminal or civil law, or to your employer through your contract of employment (Dimond, 2008). We will now look at these areas of accountability in more detail.

Professional accountability

The NMC sets the standards for professional accountability and these are laid out in a number of key documents (all available on the NMC website **www.nmc-uk.org**):

- *The Code: Standards of Conduct, Performance and Ethics for Nurses and Midwives* (NMC, 2008a);
- *Good Health and Good Character Guidance for Students, Nurses and Midwives* (NMC, 2010);
- *The Prep Handbook* (NMC, 2008b);
- *Standards for Medicines Management* (NMC, 2008c);
- *Standards to Support Learning and Assessment in Practice* (NMC, 2008d).

Further advice is also given in relation to areas such as confidentiality, accountability, consent, gifts and gratuities, clear sexual boundaries, delegation and environment of care; these provide further information on the standard of professional conduct that is required of you in exercising your professional accountability. There are also guidance documents which provide information on best practice.

Failure to adhere to the standards set by the NMC could lead to you being referred to the NMC. While the most common origin of referral is an employer followed by the police (NMC, 2009b), anyone can make a referral to the NMC where they believe that a nurse is failing to meet the standards set, or there is a concern regarding a nurse's fitness to practice. Where the NMC determines that there are grounds for a case, the nurse concerned will be referred to either the Conduct and Competence Committee or the Health Committee for adjudication. The outcome can range from no further action, a caution, conditions of practice order, suspension order to a striking-off order.

Legal accountability

Within the UK there are two legal systems: civil law and criminal law. They have different structures and different rules apply. Civil law is used to gain compensation for the injured party whereas criminal law is used to punish the person or persons who have committed an act or omission that is prohibited by law and can result in a range of penalties including fines and imprisonment.

Civil courts are usually used by a patient or their family to sue someone where they believe they have come to harm. For nurses the most likely allegations are negligence or battery (usually due to a failure to obtain consent from a patient). In civil court it would be necessary to demonstrate that the nurse is liable on a balance of probabilities.

A nurse who breaks the law will be prosecuted in a magistrates' court or crown court depending on the type of offence. In criminal law there is a higher burden of proof and the defendant has to be proven guilty beyond reasonable doubt. A memorandum of agreement exists between the NMC and the police which permits the police to share information with the NMC where a nurse is convicted of a recordable offence. Equally the NMC will inform the police where a nurse has committed a serious criminal offence and may share information with the police for other offences. A nurse who has committed a criminal offence may therefore also have to face the NMC's Conduct and Competence Committee.

Employer accountability

If you are employed you will have a contract of employment with your employer and therefore have contractual accountability to your employer. Where a nurse is believed to be in breach of their contract of employment, disciplinary processes may be invoked.

Ethical accountability

Ethical accountability 'relates to the moral requirement to be answerable to (your) patient within a practitioner/patient relationship' (Thompson et al., 2006, page 103). Ethical accountability is influenced by five ethical approaches described by Eby (2000) as:

- duty based – your professional duty to your patient;

- consequences based – focusing on consequences of actions or inaction;
- virtue based – focuses on your integrity to do the right thing;
- principle based – relates to the honesty and truthfulness of your actions;
- emotive – Eby describes this as the fear surrounding accountability.

> ## Case study: failure to follow hospital policy
>
> *John is in charge of a mental health ward on a Saturday evening. It is very busy with a number of new admissions and a client who requires close observation because of suicidal ideation. There have been a number of discussions in the ward about the use of close observation for clients following reports and articles suggesting that close observation may not necessarily prevent suicide and that the process of close observation precludes the development of a therapeutic relationship (Cutcliffe and Stevenson, 2008). In order to ensure that everyone receives a meal break and all the initial assessments for the new admissions are completed, John decides to stop close observation and implement intermittent observations. Unfortunately the client commits suicide and an investigation ensues. John is suspended from work pending the outcome of the investigation and reported to the NMC.*

In the case study a number of issues regarding John's accountability are raised. John is accountable to his employer but he failed to follow the Trust policy on close observation, which states that close observation can only be discontinued with the agreement of the client's consultant or designated deputy. John has a professional accountability to the NMC and could be referred to the Conduct and Competence Committee as failure to follow Trust procedures on close observation which led to the death of a patient could be viewed as misconduct.

The police are likely to be involved as this was a sudden death in a hospital setting and the case would become a coroner's case. The family of the client could take John to a civil court in that he failed in his duty of care to the client and therefore was deemed to be negligent.

In making the decision to stop close observation, a number of ethical issues in relation to accountability arise. John failed in his duty to his patient to ensure that he came to no harm and his integrity in making the right decision is in doubt. From a consequences viewpoint, John might argue that he considered the consequences for his staff and other clients in making the decision to reduce the level of observation.

Working within your limitations

The role of the nurse has expanded significantly in the last ten years. Nurses now take on care interventions which were once the domain of doctors, and the increasing use of technology has also changed the way that nurses work. The NMC does not specify what care interventions a nurse may or may not undertake, but the Code (NMC, 2008a) states: *You must recognise and work within the limits of your competence.* This means that if you are asked or put in a position where you are expected to undertake an activity that you do not feel competent to carry out then you must refuse to do it, explaining why. Your accountability to your employer and to the NMC means, however, that you must undertake appropriate training and learning activities not only to maintain your competence but also to develop further areas of competence that are appropriate to your area of practice. For example, if nurses regularly cannulate patients in your workplace, and it is in the best interest of the patient, then you will need to undertake training to learn this skill if it was not covered in your pre-registration nursing programme. The NMC expects all registered nurses to adjust their practice as circumstances may demand and where required to meet the changing needs of patients and clients. This may require further education and training. Increasing litigation by patients and carers has led to organisations running extensive mandatory and statutory training programmes which were discussed in Chapter 7. These will include skills training and it is important that you do not practise these skills until you have received the appropriate training. If you are unsure whether there are certain activities you should undertake there are a number of resources open to you:

- your line manager;
- your job description;
- local policies/procedures;
- NMC standards/advice/guidance documents.

If you do not feel competent to undertake any activity, then don't do it. At all times your first concern must be the safety and wellbeing of the patient.

Chapter summary

This chapter has highlighted key areas that are of key significance as you move from student to registered nurse.

This chapter has explored a range of professional issues, all of which should be familiar to you if you have recently completed a pre-registration nursing programme; however, the key difference lies in the fact that as a registered nurse the relevance of these professional issues is far more significant as you are now accountable for your actions and any omissions.

Activities: brief outline answer

Activity 12.1: What does professional behaviour look like? (page 112)

As a student you will have been expected to conduct yourself in a professional manner at all times to demonstrate that you met not only the requirements of your programme but also the standards set by the NMC in order to register as a nurse and to ensure that the trust and confidence that the public have for nurses is justified (NMC, 2009a). The NMC's *Guidance on Professional Conduct for Nursing and Midwifery Students* (NMC, 2009a) gives some insight into the professional behaviour expected of you but as Jomeen et al. (2008) point out, the NMC is not explicit in its expectations. The professional behaviours that you may have identified are:

- to follow the Code (NMC, 2008a);
- punctuality;
- appearance (adherence to dress code);
- to demonstrate good character – this covers conduct, behaviour and attitude in both your professional and personal life and would include honesty and trustworthiness, a positive attitude to

your study and practice, responding to constructive feedback, effective communication skills and adhering to the policies and procedures of both your university and the organisations where your placements took place;

- good health – to inform the university where changes in your health status may impact on your ability to deliver safe and effective practice.

Further reading

Thompson, IE, Melia, KM and Boyd, KM (2006) *Nursing Ethics*, 5th edn. Edinburgh: Churchill Livingstone.
This book takes a practical approach to both legal and ethical issues in nursing, exploring a range of topics and specialist areas

Useful websites

There are some useful scenarios on the Flying Start England website which will help you consider your professional responsibility and accountability. You will find these at: **www.flyingstartengland.nhs. uk/safe-practice**

To get you thinking about your own accountability in the workplace the Flying Start NHS website has a number of activities on this which you will find at: **www.flyingstart.scot.nhs.uk/learning-programmes/safe-practice/accountability.aspx**

The Nursing and Midwifery Council website has copies of standards and guidance that can be downloaded as well as many web pages of advice; see **www.nmc-uk.org**. You will also find it useful to read the outcomes of some of the cases referred to the NMC's Conduct and Competence Committee or the Health Committee: **www.nmc-uk.org/Hearings/Hearings-and-outcomes/**

Chapter 13
Managing risk

Chapter aims

The aim of this chapter is to explore the major elements of risk assessment and develop an understanding of implementing risk assessment and management tools within practice. At the end of this chapter you will be able to:

- identify key policies associated with risk assessment and management within the NHS;
- recognise the value of clinical governance and audit in identifying and preventing clinical risk;
- understand the implications of incident reporting and 'whistleblowing' in relation to risk management.

Introduction: assessment of risk

Throughout your professional career in the healthcare sector you will be exposed to a wide range of risk assessment and management situations. Every time healthcare services are reformed there are organisational, clinical, business and financial risks that need to be identified, assessed and controlled (Wilson and Tingle, 1999a). Given that healthcare is forever in a state of change this will require constant diligence to assess and manage risks. According to the Health Education Authority (HEA) the types of risk you will be expected to identify and manage have the potential to cause serious injuries that can have devastating consequences and can also be very costly for employers (HEA, 1997). While risk assessment is not complicated, it does require careful examination of what could cause harm to people and taking action to prevent or control that risk (HEA, 1997).

As a registered nurse you have a responsibility to minimise risk in order to maximise effective healthcare (Wilson and Tingle, 1999a). In order to do this you will need a comprehensive understanding of how to identify risks and how to minimise risks for yourself, your colleagues and those in your care.

Duty of care and risk

As a registered nurse you are accountable in law; this means that you are under a legal duty to act carefully towards patients and your colleagues. This is usually referred to as a duty of care. This is said to exist where:

- damage is foreseeable;
- there is sufficient proximity between the parties;
- it is just and reasonable to impose a duty (Hendrick, 2000).

If you do not exercise sufficient care, and as a result cause harm or injury, you may be held liable. This is called negligence. The law of negligence requires that three separate elements must be satisfied in order for a negligence claim to succeed:

- a duty of care must be owed to the claimant (the person suing for compensation);
- the defendant breeched that duty (failed to reach the standard of practice required by law);
- the damage or injury suffered was caused by that failure (Hendrick, 2010).

The point here is that as a registered nurse you are required to recognise and manage risk. Failure to do so could compromise your duty of care and lead to a claim for compensation because of your negligence.

The following activity requires you to look at a scenario and decide if a claim for negligence could be made. You will need to base your decision on the principles of duty of care.

Activity 13.1: Decision-making

Establishing duty of care

You are a newly registered nurse caring for Mrs Patel, a 77-year-old resident in a care home. Mrs Patel is frequently confused and can no longer protect herself from harm. Mrs Patel's family arrive for a visit and ask that the staff microwave is used to reheat some food the family have brought her from home. The policy in the care home states that staff must not reheat food for residents; however, you have noticed that senior staff have ignored this policy and residents' food is regularly reheated. You agree to reheat Mrs Patel's lunch and allow her family to access the staff microwave.

continued opposite...

continued...

Half an hour later you are urgently called to see Mrs Patel. You notice that her lips are swollen and she is crying. You look in her mouth and notice blisters and swelling. Her son tells you that the microwave must be faulty as the food was too hot and has scalded her mouth. He tells you that he will be suing the care home for providing faulty equipment that has harmed his mother.

What is your position in this situation?

There is a brief outline answer to this activity at the end of the chapter.

Primary liability and risk

Healthcare organisations have the responsibility to employ competent staff and provide safe equipment and premises (Lewis, 2006). This is sometimes referred to as a safe regime of care (Hendrick, 2010). This means that your organisation can be held legally responsible for organisational failure; this can include inadequate equipment, inappropriate training of staff or unsafe supervision/training (Newdick, 2005). However, this particular area of risk has significant implications as more and more areas of care are devolved to nursing responsibility (Lee, 2007). You cannot just assume that your organisation will cover all aspects of risk. For example, if you are responsible for provision of equipment or training within your organisation you will also be responsible for a failure to adequately monitor risk in these areas.

Vicarious liability and risk

In general, employers within the health service are indirectly responsible for the negligence of their employees, usually termed vicarious liability. However, your employer will usually only take responsibility for you if you are acting in their best interest (Dimond, 2008). Your employer may want to establish that your act or omission was being carried out for their benefit and this may be determined by your adherence to policy and risk procedures. From your position as a newly registered nurse it is worth considering that the law does not allow a defence of inability, lack of knowledge or inexperience (Hendrick, 2010). As a registrant it is expected that you will have the ability to recognise your limitations and take action to ensure you do not put yourself or others at risk. *The Code: Standards of Conduct, Performance and Ethics for Nurses and Midwives* (2008) states that:

- you must have the knowledge and skills for safe and effective practice when working without direct supervision;
- you must recognise and work within the limits of your competence (NMC, 2008a).

Risk and healthcare

If you are still in any doubt regarding the significance of risk assessment and management in relation to your professional role, consider the following statistics. In 2008–9 over 6,000 claims of negligence and over 3,000 claims of non-clinical negligence were made via NHS bodies and handled through the NHS Litigation Authority (NHSLA, 2010). In the period 2009–10, the NHSLA made payments totalling £827 million in respect of the five different negligence claim schemes it operates. As of March 2010 the NHSLA estimates that it has £14.9 billion of outstanding negligence claims (NHSLA, 2010). It comes as no surprise that the NHSLA incorporates an extensive risk management programme with a core aim of reducing negligent and preventable incidents in the NHS (NHSLA, 2010).

Management of risk

Most healthcare organisations providing NHS care are regularly assessed against risk management standards set by the NHSLA. There are guidelines on risk management standards for each type of healthcare organisation incorporating organisational, clinical and health and safety risks. As a result there are separate standards for the following types of healthcare providers:

- acute, PCT and independent sector standards;
- mental health and learning disability standards;
- ambulance standards;
- maternity standards (NHSLA, 2010).

As well as setting standards for risk assessment and management, the NHSLA works closely with other organisations concerned with healthcare standards and the safety of patients and healthcare workers; namely the National Patient Safety Agency (NPSA) and Quality Care Commission (QCC) (NHSLA, 2010). Both these organisations have the responsibility of identifying actual or potential risks and informing healthcare staff of actions that should be undertaken to manage that risk.

Research summary: never events

In 2008 the *High Quality Care for All – NHS Next Stage Review Final Report* (Department of Health, 2008b) proposed that a policy on 'never events' should be introduced in the NHS in England from April 2009. The NPSA was subsequently tasked with working with NHS organisations to implement the *Never Events Framework 2009/2010* (NPSA, 2009). Under this framework 'never events' were defined as serious, largely preventable patient safety incidents that should not occur if the available preventable measures have been implemented (NPSA, 2009). The core list of 'never events' includes the following:

- wrong-site surgery;
- retained instrument post-operation;
- wrong route administration of chemotherapy;
- misplaced naso or orogastric tube not detected prior to use;
- inpatient suicide using non-collapsible rails;
- escape from within the secure perimeter of medium or high secure mental health services by patients who are transferred prisoners;
- in-hospital maternal death from post-partum haemorrhage after elective caesarean section;
- intravenous administration of mis-selected concentrated potassium solution (NPSA, 2009).

Care bundles

Care bundles are becoming increasingly popular as a means of using clinical governance to ensure consistency in patient care and manage risk. They are defined as *a collection of processes needed to effectively and safely care for patients undergoing particular treatments with inherent risks. Several interventions are 'bundled' together and, when combined, significantly improve patient care outcomes* (Robb et al., 2010). Developed in the USA by the Institute for Healthcare Improvement, care bundles encourage clinical teams to examine the different interventions used for a particular disease process or care activity and use best evidence to identify a number of therapeutic interventions that together will have a significant impact on patient outcomes. For example, care bundles can be used to reduce in-hospital mortality in diverse areas such as surgical site infection, ventilator acquired pneumonia and stroke (Robb et al., 2010). Usually four to five interventions are grouped together. Importantly a care bundle focuses on how care should be delivered and *all* elements must be delivered in order for the best outcome. All healthcare professionals involved in the care of the patient group are involved in both its development and its implementation. Care bundles are audited using a simple checklist to identify whether all the interventions were implemented. Evidence of the use of care bundles has shown that it can reduce mortality (Robb et al., 2010) and reduce adverse events and complications, improving both the quality of patient care and the patient experience (NHS Modernisation Agency, 2004).

Effective risk management through clinical governance

While risk management can be seen as a tool to reduce the cost of litigation, the main aim of risk management is to reduce incidents of harm and improve the quality of care (Frith, 1999). In order to enact an effective risk management process the following factors must be in place:

- a process for identifying risks;
- an assessment and evaluation of risks;
- positive action to identify and eliminate/reduce risk (Wilson, 1999).

These three factors when incorporated into one risk assessment and management process are often given the umbrella term of 'clinical governance'. While the explicit processes that constitute clinical governance vary from one organisation to the next, there are core requirements that include processes for audit, evidence-based practice, clinical effectiveness, monitoring outcomes of care and clinical risk reduction programmes (Wilson and Tingle, 1999b).

Medicines administration

As a newly registered nurse one of the biggest immediate changes you will note to your responsibility is in relation to medicine administration. It is also one area of your professional role where you are at the greatest risk of making an error, through either an act or omission.

While administration of a medicine has inherent risks, failure to administer a medicine also poses a significant risk to patients. The National Patient Safety Agency (NPSA, 2010) highlights that doses are often omitted or delayed in hospital for a variety of reasons and that while these events may not seem serious, for some critical medicines or conditions (such as patients with sepsis or those with pulmonary embolisms) delays or omissions can cause serious harm or death. As a newly registered nurse, you may find that time pressures are putting you at risk of omitting medicines or delaying the administration time. While mistakes in medicines management are rarely deliberate, the harm done when mistakes do happen can result in significant harm or death. In fact, between September 2006 and June 2009, the NPSA received reports of 27 deaths, 68 severe harms and 21,383 other patient safety incidents relating to omitted or delayed medicines (NPSA, 2010). During your preceptorship programme it is very important that you identify areas in your professional role where you could put a patient at risk and plan ahead of time with your preceptor how to identify and eliminate these risks.

Audit

Effective auditing systems are viewed as a vital component of clinical governance (Mottram and Pickens, 2000). Audit can not only be used to identify risk but also to promote quality and thereby reduce risk (Wilson, 1999). Essentially, clinical audit involves monitoring what is being done to ensure that standards are being maintained (Maughan and Conduit, 1999). While specific areas for audit will be determined by your organisation you can be certain that your performance in certain areas will be monitored and you will be expected to monitor the performance of others. If actual or potential risk is identified this will be reported.

Reporting risk

If actual or potential risk is identified then positive action must be taken to eliminate or reduce these risks. This is often termed incident reporting and most organisations have distinct processes that all staff are expected to follow in terms of reporting risk and near-misses. A cornerstone of incident reporting involves the creation of an open, honest and blame-free organisation that values improving care, quality and getting things right (Wilson, 1999). While there are obvious benefits to reporting incidents and near-misses, it is also recognised that not all errors or risks are reported (NPSA, 2008). Very often this is put down to work pressures, not recognising risks or fear of blame (NPSA, 2008). As a newly registered nurse you may find all of these factors are influential on your decision-making when it comes to reporting of actual or potential risks. However, you must remember that as a registered nurse you now have a professional duty of care to not only take an active role in clinical governance but also to report incidents and near-misses. To not do this would be seen as a breech in your duty of care. For this reason it is imperative that you familiarise yourself not only with current risk policy in your organisation, but also with the processes in place in your organisation with regard to:

- incident reporting;
- safeguarding;
- whistleblowing;
- raising concern.

Case study: Sean speaks about reporting an incident

In my second month of being a registered nurse I put up an IV infusion on a patient that was meant to run over eight hours and somehow I got it totally wrong and the whole litre of saline went in over four hours. No one else noticed what had happened and my first reaction was to wonder if I could cover it up. It sounds terrible but I was in such a panic wondering what my manager would think of me when I told them and also I had this crazy thought that I might get sacked. I guess for a few seconds I was tempted just to pretend it hadn't happened. That probably says a lot about the pressure I was under more than anything. Anyway, I did come clean, mainly because I was really worried about the patient. I'm so relieved that I did that because it taught me what it really meant to be a nurse. My manager praised me for being honest and professional and she talked me through reporting it to a doctor so the patient could be monitored properly. We sat down and did the incident report together and she made me realise that even though an error had happened it wasn't the end. She just got me to look at what I had done in a really constructive way so we could stop a similar thing happening again. In the end all that happened was I learnt to be a better nurse.

Activity 13.2: Leadership and management

Incident reporting

Take some time now to familiarise yourself with the processes involved in incident reporting within your organisation. You may want to access specific policies that relate to incident reporting or perhaps speak with your preceptor regarding the required processes. In particular, you should take some time to consider the following:

- What method of incident reporting is used (computerised reporting, paper reporting, or both)?
- What types of incidents am I required to report?
- What happens to my report?

As this activity is based on your own research, there is no outline answer at the end of the chapter.

Whistleblowing

There may be a time during your professional career when you witness others involved in incidents or situations or practices that give you cause for concern. The NMC takes a very clear position in terms of your role and responsibility regarding risk. *The Code: Standards of Conduct, Performance and Ethics for Nurses and Midwives* (2008a) outlines the following.

- *You must act without delay if you believe that you, a colleague or anyone else may be putting someone at risk.*
- *You must inform someone in authority if you experience problems that prevent you working within this code or other nationally agreed standards.*
- *You must report your concerns in writing if problems in the environment of care are putting people at risk.*
- *As a professional, you are personally accountable for actions and omissions in your practice, and must be able to justify your decisions* (NMC, 2008a).

You will notice that your relationship with risk assessment and management is an active rather than a passive role. In other words, you are expected to act on the possibility of risk rather than act once an incident has occurred. The NMC does not differentiate either between risk to patients, and risk to yourself or colleagues. All areas of potential risk are covered as part of your professional responsibility and are deemed of equal importance.

Reporting concerns, whether they are about an individual or practices within an organisation, is often referred to as whistleblowing. Of course, just because it is part of your professional role does not make whistleblowing any easier or more palatable to do. Research undertaken by the NPSA (2008) indicates that for staff to feel comfortable to report incidents there must be five key elements in place:

- individual reporters must get feedback;
- there must be a focus on learning rather than blame;
- frontline staff must be trained in incident reporting;
- it must be easy to report;
- individual staff must feel that reporting matters (NPSA, 2008).

For this reason, most organisations have now adopted specific guidelines on incident reporting that address each of these areas, with advice on escalating concerns within the organisation. You should take the time to familiarise yourself with such guidance for your current organisation and also look at the NMC's publication *Raising and Escalating Concerns: Guidance for Nurses and Midwives* (NMC, 2010c), which provides guidance on the steps to follow where you have concerns regarding the safety or wellbeing of the public, which may include:

- *danger or risk to health and safety, such as health and safety violations;*
- *issues regarding staff conduct, such as unprofessional attitudes or behaviour, including concerns related to equality and diversity;*
- *issues regarding care delivery involving nurses, midwives or other staff members;*
- *issues related to the environment of care in the broadest sense, such as resources, products, people, staffing or organisation-wide concerns;*
- *issues related to the health of a colleague, which may affect their ability to practise safely;*
- *misuse or unavailability of clinical equipment, including a lack of adequate training;*
- *financial malpractice, including criminal acts and fraud* (NMC, 2010c, page 5).

The consequences of failures to report concerns were highlighted in the investigation into Mid Staffordshire NHS Foundation Trust undertaken by the then Healthcare Commission (now the Care Quality Commission) in March 2009. The investigation was triggered following analysis of mortality rates in England, which found that the Trust had high mortality rates for patients admitted as emergencies. The investigation and inquiries that followed found serious failings in the quality of care with even the most basic elements of patient care neglected.

In his review of the lessons to be learnt from the investigation, Dr David Colin-Thomé said: *What has particularly shocked and disappointed me is that no NHS organisations, staff or representatives of the public reported any serious concerns about emergency services in the hospital* (2009, page 3).

Chapter summary

Throughout this chapter we have explored issues associated with risk assessment and explored the processes for implementing risk assessment and management tools within practice. There has been an opportunity to understand the implications of incident reporting and whistleblowing in relation to risk management, including professional implications. As the various roles and responsibilities of nurses change, so will the requirement to identify your role in relation to risk assessment and management.
As your career develops so will the expectation that you become more active in the implementation of clinical governance and audit systems to identify and prevent clinical risk.

Activities: brief outline answer

Activity 13.1: Establishing duty of care (page 120)

This activity required you to look at a scenario and decide if a claim for negligence could be made based on the principles of duty of care.

In this situation a claim for negligence could be made; however, this claim would be made against you rather than your organisation. In law, you would be seen to have a duty of care to Mrs Patel by nature of the nurse/patient relationship. You will have breeched that duty of care by failing to protect her from harm. Forseeability that food reheated in the staff microwave may cause a patient harm has already been established by your organisation. For this reason the policy of the organisation was to not allow reheating of food. By ignoring this policy you were not acting in your employer's best interest and would not be covered under vicarious liability. The scalding to Mrs Patel's mouth would be seen as a result of your negligence.

Further reading

Frances, R (2010) *Independent Inquiry into Care Provided by Mid Staffordshire NHS Foundation Trust January 2005–March 2009*, Volumes 1 and 2. London: The Stationery Office.
This lengthy report provides a salutary lesson about the consequences of poor governance and failure to listen to staff and patient concerns.

Useful websites

Public Concern at Work (PCaW): **www.pcaw.co.uk**
An independent whistleblowing charity.

National Patient Safety Agency: **www.npsa.nhs.uk**
Provides useful information regarding patient safety issues.

There are some useful web resources on clinical governance on the Flying Start NHS website. You can access these links via: **www.flyingstart.scot.nhs.uk/learning-programmes/safe-practice/clinical-governance.aspx**

The 'Managing risk' section on the Flying Start England website has a range of resources that will be useful to explore this topic further. You can access these resources at: **www.flyingstartengland.nhs. uk/safepractice/managingrisk**

Chapter 14
Equality and diversity

Preceptorship Framework and KSF

This chapter maps to the following elements of the Department of Health Preceptorship Framework and the NHS Knowledge and Skills Framework.

Preceptorship Framework
- Equality and diversity
- Develop confidence and self-awareness
- Understand policies and procedures
- Implement the Code and professional values

NHS Knowledge and Skills Framework
- Equality and diversity
- Communication
- Personal and people development
- Service improvement
- Quality

Chapter aims

The aim of this chapter is to gain an understanding of equality and diversity issues within healthcare and how these relate to your professional role. At the end of this chapter you will be able to:

- identify the key elements of equality and diversity;
- understand the principles for managing a range of equality and diversity issues within an organisation;
- explore the relevance of equality and diversity in relation to care of patients and your membership within an organisation.

Introduction: understanding equality and diversity

While the majority of people would support the need for equality and diversity to be a fundamental approach within a healthcare organisation, very few people would be confident to expand on the legislation that governs equality and diversity issues. For others, their knowledge of equality and diversity is out of date or misconstrued. As a result, it is often the case that healthcare providers have a poor understanding of their role in promoting good practice in relation to equality and diversity. All too often, issues related to equality and diversity are misrepresented and subject to myth and false assumptions within healthcare organisations. As a registered nurse it is expected that you not only have a thorough grasp of issues related to equality and diversity but that you actively promote and defend good practice in relation to equality and diversity. You can be sure that for the remainder of your nursing career it will be a core requirement of your professional role.

The origins of equality

Before we go any further we will need to understand exactly what it is that we mean by equality and diversity. Let's start with dispelling the myth that issues related to equality and diversity are new or only being talked about in recent years. Have a look at the following excerpt from *The Unanimous Declaration of the Thirteen United States of America*:

> *We hold these truths to be self-evident, that all men are created equal, that they are endowed by their Creator with certain unalienable Rights, that among these are Life, Liberty and the pursuit of Happiness.* (USHistory.org, 2010)

In the very famous opening sentence of what is commonly referred to as the American Declaration of Independence is a statement that addresses the subject of equality. As it is widely accepted that this declaration was made in 1776, we can easily confirm that issues of equality and diversity are neither new or of recent importance. What is true, however, is that we have come a long way and have made significant progress in relation to defining what equality really is and how diversity relates to equality.

You may have noticed a major flaw in this declaration, namely that all men are created equal. That is quite clearly incorrect. We know without any dispute that in fact we are all very different from each other; we are not at all equal, as evidenced by our unique genetic makeup. In recent years this uniqueness has been explained under the term 'diversity'. In this way we are able to account for our differences by agreeing that we all have equal *value* rather than are all the same.

Of course, the second immediate flaw is that the declaration makes no reference to women, and by the standards we are familiar with today this would be totally unacceptable. However, at the time the declaration was written, 'men' was generally accepted to mean 'people'; the use of inclusive language is a relatively new addition to our current dialogue. However, while the language may be outdated and not based on our current scientific understanding, the desire of the writing does still resonate today. There is a clear intention here that all people should be treated as having equal value. In recent years we have recognised this understanding as equality and diversity.

Equality and diversity in patient care

One of the key elements of equality and diversity is often referred to as cultural competence. As a registered nurse this means that unless you are able to take into account the social and cultural worlds of your patients you will not be fulfilling the requirements of professional practice. These are the core components of cultural competence:

- acceptance of differences as normal, and only to be expected, for human beings;
- acceptance of the inherent right of all residents in a society to identify as part of the society and acceptance of the resultant changes (Baxter, 2001).

To begin this process it is necessary that you have a very clear understanding of the range of social and cultural backgrounds of the patients you will be caring for.

Diversity and the NMC

Without an understanding of cultural competence you will be failing in your duty of care to patients. As we covered this extensively in Chapter 13 there is no need to cover duty of care again. However, it is important to grasp the link between cultural competence and *The Code: Standards of Conduct, Performance and Ethics for Nurses and Midwives* (2008a). The following statements within the Code make your position as a registrant very clear:

- You must demonstrate a personal and professional commitment to equality and diversity.
- You must treat people as individuals and respect their dignity.
- You must not discriminate in any way against those in your care (NMC, 2008a).

This means that in order to ensure cultural competence you must at all times be aware of the diverse needs of the patient population you are caring for. Without this knowledge you may well be inadvertently failing in your duty to care for someone as an individual, perhaps making assumptions regarding their care wishes or personal preferences.

Case study: assumptions in equality and diversity

Stan is being admitted to the ward and Jenny, his nurse, notices a ring on his wedding finger. Based on this information she makes the following assumptions:

- *Stan is heterosexual;*
- *Stan is married;*
- *Stan is in contact with his wife;*
- *Stan wants his wife to be his contact person.*

Based on these assumptions Jenny asks for his wife's contact details. She shows obvious surprise when Stan states that he is homosexual and provides the nurse with the contact details of his husband. Jenny has learnt a valuable lesson in equality and diversity. Rather than assuming that Stan is heterosexual, married and in contact with his wife she should have asked him who he preferred as a contact person and asked what the nature of the relationship was. This would give Stan the freedom to disclose as much or as little as he wishes to and still ensure that care can be provided.

In the case study above, Jenny has not shown the degree of cultural competence expected of a registered nurse. She has made many assumptions and as a result, Stan has been forced to disclose information about his personal life in order to prevent further assumptions regarding his care needs. As a newly registered nurse you will have already been exposed to a range of equality and diversity issues throughout your education. However, now that you are a registrant it will be up to you to ensure that you remain culturally aware and competent in the care you deliver. Unless you have an understanding of what this is, you run a very high risk of making unintended errors.

Activity 14.1: Evidence-based practice and research

Investigating diversity

This activity will help you to understand the diversity of the social and cultural backgrounds of the patients you care for in your organisation. While diversity can be related to multiple areas it is useful to categorise diversity into separate themes. These can include any of the following:

- age;
- ability and disability;
- gender;
- race;
- religion or belief;
- sexual orientation.

Use this list to ascertain the diversity of the population you care for. For example, you could focus on the age distribution of your clients, or the different ethnic or religious groups represented in your practice area. As this may be quite a major undertaking you could choose a specific area to audit, perhaps just the current inpatients on one day or a random selection of clients that may attend or be linked to your clinic.

As this is a reflective activity, there is no outline answer at the end of this chapter.

By completing Activity 14.1 it should become very clear that there is no such thing as a 'typical patient'. Every single patient you provide care for as a nurse will have a unique set of needs that you must be aware of and conversant with in order to provide nursing care. It will also become clear that you will not be able to make assumptions or infer care requirements based on how someone looks or the way they speak.

Case study: Robert speaks of his experience as a patient

Last year I had to move from London to Bristol. This meant I had to change GP so I went to a health assessment for new patients run by the practice nurse. My mum and dad are both Nigerian and came to the UK in the 1950s. I was born in London and I consider myself to be Black British; I'm really proud to say that. Anyway this practice nurse took one look at me and said 'It's a lot colder here than where you were you born'. I said 'Not really, Bristol has about the same weather as London'. She was so surprised and she told me she was born in Guyana and had assumed I was Nigerian. In reality she had assumed she knew me based on how I looked and had obviously got it really wrong. We laughed about it and that was that but it made me realise that people probably assume things about me all the time that aren't right. Mind you, I probably assume things about them too.

Equality and diversity in organisations

Of course, the issues of equality and diversity do not apply only to patient care. Equality and diversity considerations will be a major part of your working relationships, in terms of both how the organisation responds to you and how you respond to the organisation. The NHS Constitution highlights clear aspirations for equality and diversity which include the following elements:

- a comprehensive service for all;
- equal access dignity and respect for patients and staff (NHS Employers, 2009).

In addition, the Equality Act (2010) now provides a revised legislative framework with an aim of protecting the rights of individuals and to advance equality of opportunity for all. The Equality Act has updated, simplified and strengthened all previous legislation. The key aim of this Equality Act is therefore to ensure a simple, modern and accessible framework of discrimination law that not only protects individuals from unfair treatment but also promotes a fair and more equal society (Equality Act, 2010).

Research summary: the Equality Act

The Equality Act 2010 came into force on 1 October 2010. The major features of the Equality Act 2010 at the point of implementation include:

- the basic framework of protection against direct and indirect discrimination, harassment and victimisation in services and public functions; premises; work; education; associations; and transport;
- changing the definition of gender reassignment, by removing the requirement for medical supervision;
- levelling up protection for people discriminated against because they are perceived to have, or are associated with someone who has, a protected characteristic, so providing new protection for people like carers;
- clearer protection for breastfeeding mothers;
- applying the European definition of indirect discrimination to all protected characteristics;
- extending protection from indirect discrimination to disability;
- introducing a new concept of 'discrimination arising from disability', to replace protection under previous legislation lost as a result of a legal judgment.
- applying the detriment model to victimisation protection (aligning with the approach in employment law);
- harmonising the thresholds for the duty to make reasonable adjustments for disabled people;
- extending protection from third party harassment to all protected characteristics.
- making it more difficult for disabled people to be unfairly screened out when applying for jobs, by restricting the circumstances in which employers can ask job applicants questions about disability or health;

continued overleaf...

continued...

- allowing claims for direct gender pay discrimination where there is no actual comparator;
- making pay secrecy clauses unenforceable;
- extending protection in private clubs to sex, religion or belief, pregnancy and maternity, and gender reassignment;
- introducing new powers for employment tribunals to make recommendations which benefit the wider workforce;
- harmonising provisions allowing voluntary positive action (Equality Act, 2010).

Equality and diversity in patient care

The Equality Act has implications in the care that you deliver and the services that you provide for those under your care. For example, the NHS has made a commitment to providing same-sex accommodation for all patients in all hospitals. Recognition that mixed-sex hospital accommodation can be difficult for some patients for a variety of personal and cultural reasons, the NHS has set an agenda to treat all patients in privacy and with dignity. All hospital Trusts are therefore required to provide same-sex accommodation for all patients (NHS Choices, 2010). As this is very difficult to achieve in some care settings, for example ITU, recovery and day care units it is worth finding out the specific policy for same-sex accommodation your organisation has adopted.

As a registrant you will of course be expected to comply with policies that promote equality and diversity, with the requirement for same-sex accommodation being just one example. Not only will this require you to understand the various local policies that promote equality and diversity in your workplace, but also that you identify areas where cultural competence may be at risk and take action to rectify these situations.

Activity 14.2: Evidence-based practice and research

Equality and diversity in patient care

Take some time to investigate the various aspects of patient/client care that require you to be culturally competent. For example, are patients able to select food from a menu that caters for their cultural or religious preferences? Are interpreting services displayed in areas where staff and clients can review their options and make an informed choice? You may like to look at one specific area and then identify if current policies are inclusive to all service users or discriminate against specific groups of services users. If you do highlight any areas that require attention, what will you do?

There is a brief outline answer at the end of the chapter.

Political correctness

In recent years the term 'politically correct' has gained notoriety and is now commonly referred to in a negative context. You may have heard references to political correctness in terms of it 'going mad'. In fact, political correctness has now become an unfortunate euphemism for any act or policy that is associated with equality and diversity and is seen as irrational. What has been forgotten is the basis of 'politically correct' language, which aims to ensure that communication in the workplace is free from discrimination, intimidation, harassment and stereotyping. It is important to remember that, very often, language or behaviours can be used to create an atmosphere of bias. Some examples are provided in the following scenarios.

Scenario 1

John is a staff nurse on a care of the elderly ward. When patients who require assistance with moving from a bed to a chair are inpatients, John is frequently asked to assist with the transfer. He realises that he is being asked more than other staff members to assist because he is male.

Scenario 2

Julie is a manager of three learning disability group homes. The staff in these homes come from a wide range of culturally diverse backgrounds. Some of her staff identify as Hindu, others identify as Christian. It is common practice for staff who identify as Hindu to request days off over Divali, and those who identify as Christian to request days off over Christmas. When a new member of staff joins the team Julie assumes that as her ethnic origin is Asian, she will also request time off over the Divali festival. When Julie states this she offends her new employee, who actually identifies as Christian.

The above scenarios demonstrate that while actions and language may not be illegal, they can be used to imply a bias that does not support equality or diversity. In this respect, incorrect use of language and actions can be highly offensive and is at odds with your professional role. In addition, failure to adhere to good practice guidelines in relation to equality and diversity results in wasted time and resources. Equality within an organisation helps with quality of staff recruitment, professional development of all staff and the quality of services being delivered (Blakemore, 2009).

Chapter summary

In reading this chapter you should now have a greater understanding of current equality and diversity issues within healthcare and how these relate to your professional role. While it is important to understand the key legislation that underpins equality and diversity, the real relevance is how equality and diversity issues will impact on the care of patients and your membership within any healthcare organisation. This chapter has highlighted that maintaining good practice in terms of equality and diversity is not just the responsibility of senior management, it applies to everyone within an organisation, at every level, and at every stage of their career. As a newly qualified nurse it will be expected that you take an active role in promoting fairness and equality of opportunity and tackle disadvantage and discrimination through your work practices on a daily basis.

Activities: brief outline answer

Activity 14.2: Equality and diversity in patient care (page 134)

Very often cultural competence is not considered in terms of planning or facilitating patient care. Yet in order to achieve holistic care, awareness of the individual needs of the whole person will be a core element. Consider the services your organisation provides to meet the spiritual or religious requirements of service users. Are there designated quiet rooms, chapels, prayer rooms or multifaith rooms? Are there washing facilities? Most importantly, are there any obvious areas of discrimination or bias? If so, what can be done to ensure equality and diversity is promoted?

Further reading

Hunt, B (2007) Managing equality and cultural diversity in the health workforce. *Journal of Clinical Nursing,*16: 2252–59.
This article explores some very practical and sensitive issues related to the support of overseas trained nurses as they enter the health workforce in the UK.

Useful websites

If you would like to review your knowledge of different cultural and religious beliefs you may find the multi-faith resource activity useful. You can find this activity at: **www.flyingstartengland.nhs.uk/ equality-and-diversity/diversity**

There are clear links between equality and diversity and patient autonomy. To explore these links you could explore the various activities in the patient autonomy section of the Flying Start NHS website. You can find these resources at: **www.flyingstart.scot.nhs.uk/learning-programmes/equality-and-diversity/patient-autonomy.aspx**

Chapter 15
Decision-making

Chapter aims

The aim of this chapter is to explore decision-making in the context of clinical practice. By the end of this chapter you will be able to:

- understand the importance of problem-solving and decision-making within clinical practice;
- consider different approaches to problem-solving and decision-making;
- identify the sources of information or knowledge that you can use to help you make decisions;
- appreciate the importance of shared decision-making and the nurse's role in supporting patients through the decision-making process.

Introduction

We all make decisions every day; however, as a nurse the decisions you make in clinical practice could have significant repercussions for patients and clients, yourself and other healthcare professionals, particularly if they are the wrong ones. Healthcare is becoming increasingly more complex and the sheer pace of change and the volume of information with which we are confronted make it a challenge to keep up-to-date with best practice and policy in order to ensure the best outcomes for your patients and clients. It is important, therefore, that you recognise when you need help in making a decision. While there will be an expectation that as a registered nurse you are capable of safe and effective care without being supervised, that does not mean that you are expected to know the answer to everything. There will be times when you are unsure what the best course of action is, and at these times it is important you seek advice from other colleagues or access information from appropriate sources. As a registered nurse you are professionally accountable for your actions, which means that the decisions you make must be based on sound evidence. This chapter will look at the theories underpinning decision-making, the resources available to you and the importance of involving patients in the decision-making process.

Decision-making, clinical judgement and problem-solving

There is a tendency for decision-making, clinical judgement and problem-solving to be used interchangeably; but they are different (Sullivan et al., 2010). While the problem-solving process is used to solve a problem, the decision-making process may not always involve a problem, just a number of options. Clinical judgement, on the other hand, is used to guide decision-making through the assessment and evaluation of both objective and subjective data about a patient. For example, making a judgement about whether a patient is at risk of falling will lead to a decision as to whether any interventions are required to reduce that risk. Standing (2010) provides a lengthy and detailed definition for clinical decision-making developed from her doctoral research, in which she identifies the skills required as well as the nurse's role as a decision-maker:

> *Clinical decision-making is a complex process involving observation, information processing, critical thinking, evaluating evidence, applying relevant knowledge, problem solving skills, reflection and clinical judgement to select the best course of action which optimizes a patient's health and minimizes any harm. The role of the clinical decision-maker in nursing is, therefore, to be professionally accountable for accurately assessing a patient's needs using appropriate sources of information, and planning nursing interventions that address problems and which they are competent to perform*
> (Standing, 2005, page 34).

Activity 15.1: Reflective decision-making

Your decision-making

Consider a clinical decision you have made recently. What was the decision about? What judgements led you to that decision?

As this is a reflective activity, there is no outline answer at the end of this chapter.

Thompson and Dowding (2009) identified 11 different types of decisions made by nurses (Table 15.1) and the range of different decision types demonstrate the range and complexity of decision-making by nurses. Can you see where the decision you described in Activity 15.1 fits?

Assessment	Deciding to undertake an assessment or to use a specific assessment tool
Diagnosis	Making a decision based on a collection of signs and symptoms
Intervention/effectiveness	Choosing between two or more potential interventions
Targeting (a subcategory of intervention)	Deciding which patient/client group will benefit best from a specific intervention
Prevention (a subcategory of intervention)	Choosing which intervention may prevent specific health outcomes
Timing (a subcategory of intervention)	Deciding when the best time is to implement an intervention
Referral	Deciding whom to refer a client or patient to for care or management
Communication	Deciding how best to deliver or receive information to or from clients and/or their family
Information seeking	Deciding whether or not to seek information further from another source (e.g. patient/carer/colleague/research)
Service organisation, delivery and management	Deciding which approach to take in organising delivery or managing a service
Experiential, understanding or hermeneutic	Using cues to make a decision as to how another may be experiencing an event

Table 15.1: Decision types made by nurses
Source: adapted from Thompson and Dowding (2009)

Factors that influence decision-making

There are a range of factors that will influence the decisions you make, including:

- knowledge;
- previous experience;
- self-confidence;
- ethical codes;
- personal values;
- patient/client choice;
- legislation;
- environmental stressors – time, staffing, resources.

Previous experience was identified by Benner (1984) as essential for developing expertise in clinical judgements (see Research summary below). Lack of self-confidence, which is often seen in the newly registered nurse, can prevent an individual from making decisions in case they may be wrong, which is further influenced by concerns regarding their accountability. Ethical codes and personal values will influence where a person's attention is directed, and so influence the options chosen. Where the patient has been involved in the decision-making process, their choice will determine the actions to be taken (or not taken, if that is their choice). The law (e.g. health and safety regulations) may limit the choices open to you, or require specific actions to be taken. Environmental stressors can also impact on your decision-making: lack of time, staff or resources may limit the options open to you or can impact on the quality of your decision-making.

Activity 15.2: Reflective decision-making

Factors influencing decision-making

Consider again the clinical decision you identified in Activity 15.1. What factors influenced your decision?

As this is a reflective activity, there is no outline answer at the end of this chapter.

Research summary: Benner's *From Novice to Expert*

Benner's (1984) seminal work, which looked at the skill acquisition and clinical judgements by senior nursing students, newly graduated nurses and experienced nurses, was conducted between 1978 and 1981. Healthcare has changed significantly since this research was undertaken, with a significant increase in the amount and calibre of nursing research being published providing a large evidence base which nurses can use to inform their actions. However, Benner's findings still resonate with today's nurses and her model continues to be used by nurse educators and practitioners.

Benner used interviews and participant observation in order to clarify and describe the different characteristics of nurses at different stages of their education and practice and, using the Dreyfus model of skill acquisition, identified five stages from novice nurse to expert practitioner:

- The novice stage – this relates to the student nurse who has no experience of an area of practice and therefore is taught rules to enable them to perform safely in practice. The rules are general in nature to enable them to be applied to any context: as a consequence the student nurse's behaviour is limited and inflexible.
- Advanced beginner (new graduate) – the nurse is starting to build up experiences that can be used to develop principles to guide actions. The advanced beginner is very aware of their accountability and professional responsibility but still requires some help in identifying priorities and still sees situations in their component parts.
- Competent stage (one to two years in practice) – the nurse is able to set priorities, developing critical thinking skills, and is able to predict immediate possible events based on past experience and so better plan for patient needs.

continued opposite...

continued...

- Proficiency – the nurse sees situations as wholes rather than parts and using past experience is able to predict what the expected events will be for the patient but is able to recognise when the expected doesn't happen. The proficient nurse uses 'maxims' for guidance and is able to adapt to changing situations.
- Expert – the nurse no longer relies on rules, guidelines or maxims but has an intuitive grasp of the whole, although will fall back on the use of analytical approaches in new situations or where problems occur.

Whilst the model describes a progressive development linked with experience, a nurse who moves from one area of practice to another (e.g. inpatient nursing to community) may move from a higher level to a lower level until experience is gained in that new area of practice.

Case study: the advanced beginner and the expert nurse

John is an 80-year-old patient who was admitted during the night with a chest infection. At handover, the night shift inform the day shift that John has been very restless and keeps getting out of bed and pacing round the ward. He won't keep his oxygen mask on, which they feel is contributing to his confusion and restlessness.

Sarah is a recently qualified nurse and John is one of the patients allocated to her for the day. She checks on John and finds him walking round the bay so asks him to return to his seat and places his oxygen mask back on his face. She takes a set of observations which show his respiratory and pulse rate are slightly raised, and his oxygen saturations are at the lower side of normal. During the course of the morning she has to repeatedly return to John to ask him to sit down and replace his oxygen mask and starts to feel quite stressed as he won't comply with her requests to stay by his bed and she is concerned he may fall or come to harm.

Jose has been working on the ward for five years and sees John walking round the ward. She joins him and guides him back to his bed, talking to him as they go. Her immediate impression is that John is well-orientated and shows no signs of confusion. She undertakes a set of observations which are similar to the ones that Sarah took but acceptable given that he has been walking up and down the ward. She also looks at his colour – he is pink and well perfused. She asks him a few more questions to try to determine how orientated he is to time and place and he is able to answer all the questions correctly. At this point Jose intuitively grasps that John's restlessness may be due to other reasons that have not been explored and sits down to talk to him further. Through further questioning she elicits that he had been given sedation during the night but is frightened of falling asleep in case he doesn't wake up so is walking up and down the ward to keep himself awake. Jose explores further his fear of not waking up should he fall asleep and is able to reassure him that this will not happen and that she will keep a close eye on him while he rests.

In the case study Sarah has followed the directions for John's care regarding observations and oxygen therapy and accepted the night nurse's diagnosis that John is confused, assuming his raised respiratory and pulse rate were due to hypoxia. She has not considered other options for his restlessness. Her main concern has been her accountability should John come to harm. Jose, however, looked at the whole picture and intuitively grasped that neither John's behaviour nor his clinical observations were representative of a confused or hypoxic patient and sought more information to help her make an informed decision. As an expert practitioner, Jose was open to other possibilities which Sarah hadn't considered.

Decision-making models

There are three commonly accepted approaches to decision-making: information processing, intuitive-humanistic approaches and cognitive continuum theory, which combines both the former approaches (Muir, 2004; Standing, 2010; Thompson and Dowding, 2002). We will now look at each of these approaches.

Information processing

The information processing model recognises that humans store information in both their short term and long term memories. Information stored within the short term memory is used to trigger retrieval of relevant information from the long term memory. So, for example, having met a patient and undertaken an initial assessment, the information you have gained from that assessment will reside in your short term memory. This new information will then trigger retrieval of relevant information from your long term memory. This information may have been stored there from previous admissions and theoretical learning you have undertaken and will enable you to make judgements about the patient, explanations as to why the patient may be exhibiting certain signs and symptoms or behaving in a certain way. This may result in a number of explanations, and preference will be given to the one supported by the greatest evidence. The information processing approach is one that tends to be more widely used by the less experienced nurse but the ability to generate multiple explanations will depend on the nurse's knowledge base and previous experience. Information processing is an analytical approach to decision-making.

Intuitive–humanistic approach

Intuition is described by Benner and Tanner (1987) as *understanding without a rationale* (page 23) and is an approach that is commonly accepted as being used by the expert nurse (Benner, 1984). Intuitive decision-making involves seeing the whole picture rather than breaking down a situation into its component parts (the analytical, information processing approach) so is a more rapid approach to decision-making and is closely linked to Schon's (1987) reflection in action. The nurse, through a wealth of experience of previous cases, which may be similar, and the knowledge that has been developed over years of practice, is able to see patterns and reject those that don't fit at a subconscious level and come to a decision about the patient's diagnosis or the interventions required.

Cognitive continuum theory

Cognitive continuum theory (Hammond, 1996) recognises that humans use a range of decision-making processes and fits well with the decision-making that takes place in healthcare. Standing

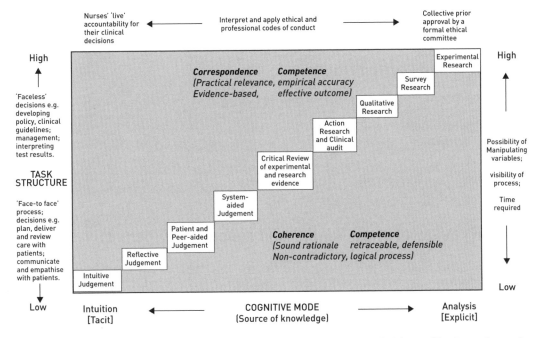

Figure 15.1: Standing's revised cognitive continuum of clinical judgement and decision-making in nursing – nine modes of justice (from Standing, 2008, page 130).

(2008) revised cognitive continuum theory to make it more applicable to nursing (Figure 15.1). The model shows nine modes of practice; from intuitive judgement at one end to the highly structured experimental research at the other end.

The type of judgement that a person will use in a particular situation will depend on a number of factors, including:

- the structure of the task in hand – the less structured a task, and more practical and personal it is, the more the judgement used will be towards the intuitive end of the continuum;
- the time available – the more time available, the more the judgement can be made at the analytical end of the continuum.

The revised model not only offers nurses an opportunity to consider the different approaches to decision-making that they can use, but also recognises the importance of involving the patient in decision-making.

Resources for decision-making

Standing's (2008) model also gives pointers to resources for making decisions.

Patient and peer judgement

Colleagues are probably the first resource that you are likely to use and many patients can equally be a valuable resource, particularly patients with long term conditions who are usually well-informed about their health status and treatments. In some cases it will be inappropriate for a single person to make a decision and in those situations decision-making will take place through discussion of the relevant members of the multidisciplinary team with (it is hoped) the patient at the centre of the discussion.

System-aided judgement

This includes use of:

* validated assessment tools;
* clinical guidelines;
* protocols;
* problem-solving frameworks;
* computerised decision analysis systems.

Critical review of experiential and research evidence

There is a wealth of research evidence available that can aid the decision-making process and ensure an evidence-based approach to care is taken. However, you need to have effective critical appraisal skills in order to sift out research which is sound from that which is not. This resource will be used where an immediate decision is not required.

Action research and clinical audit, qualitative research, survey research and experimental research are the remaining four modes of research described by Standing. You can either utilise published results from one or more of these approaches to help make an informed decision, or undertake action research, clinical audit or a research study to answer a question you have that does not require an immediate response.

Shared decision-making

The principle at the centre of the white paper *Equity and Excellence: Liberating the NHS* (Department of Health, 2010b) is *no decision about me without me* (page 3). The aim of the proposals set out in the paper is to empower patients to share in the decisions about their care. Unfortunately, evidence suggests that shared decision-making has not been widely adopted in practice to date (Légaré et al., 2010), with O'Grady and Jadad (2010) identifying time constraints as being a particular barrier. The sheer volume of information available to patients, particularly via the internet, and the opportunities available for patients to share experiences via discussion forums, social networking sites and mailing lists (O'Grady and Jadad, 2010), means that patients today are far better informed than in the past and are able to take a more active part in the decision-making process. Shared decision-making is at the hub of patient-centred care and congruent with nursing values, and therefore should be an aspect of patient care with which nurses feel very comfortable. Makoul (2006) identified eight essential elements that should be included during a consultation between a healthcare professional and a patient which Légaré et al. (2010) summarised as:

* *define/explain the healthcare problem;*
* *present options;*
* *discuss pros/cons (benefits/risks/costs);*
* *clarify patient values/preferences;*

- *discuss patient ability/self-efficacy;*
- *present what is known and make recommendations;*
- *check/clarify the patient's understanding;*
- *make or explicitly defer a decision;*
- *arrange follow up* (page 3).

As a newly registered nurse you may feel that you don't have the experience and/or knowledge to support patients with decision-making. However, although the focus on shared decision-making has been on medical treatments and interventions, you should be involving patients in decision-making around nursing care interventions and lifestyle choices as well as advocating for the patient in situations where other healthcare professionals are not offering the opportunity for shared decision-making.

Patient decision aids (PDAs)

Whilst you may not feel confident with being involved in shared decision-making at the moment, there are a range of tools that patients can use, which you can provide for your patients, or else point them in the right direction where they are web-based. PDA is a term used to describe a range of tools which prepare patients to make a decision based on evidence, regarding treatments or screening by providing them with:

- up-to-date information based on best evidence on the different options and the likely outcomes for each (this information can be designed for the healthcare professional to inform the patient and/or be specifically aimed at the patient);
- an exploration of values and what is important to them (e.g. length of life versus quality of life);
- support from a healthcare professional in deciding between the different options (National Steering Group for Decision Support Aids in Urology, 2005).

PDAs usually include one or more of the following:

- information leaflets that include options with benefits, risks and costs for each;
- videos;
- values clarification exercises to enable patients to identify their own values;
- patient stories of their own experiences with different interventions;
- questionnaires to help patients clarify their treatment preference;
- guides that the patient can use to help them ask the right questions when meeting with a healthcare professional.

PDAs are useful tools not only for you to use to help a patient with the decision-making process, but also to help you develop your knowledge and understanding of specific health issues.

Activity 15.3: Evidence-based practice and research

Identify patient decision aids
Are PDAs used in your area of practice? If not, explore what PDAs may be available that are relevant to your area and share these with colleagues. There are a range of websites that identify PDAs, which is a useful starting point.

As this is an activity specific to your area of practice, there is no outline answer at the end of this chapter.

Evaluating the effectiveness of decision-making

While it is not appropriate to evaluate every decision you make, it is important that you pause at times to review whether the decision you made is the right one, especially where the outcomes are not as expected or you had a degree of uncertainty about the decision. There are a range of methods you can use to do this, including:

- reflective practice;
- peer review and feedback;
- clinical supervision.

During your preceptorship period you will have access to your preceptor, who is likely to be your first point of contact in reviewing a decision you have made and can help you reflect on the steps you took in making that decision. A reflective diary is a useful tool to record decisions made and reflections on the outcomes from them; you can then use the diary as a prompt when meeting with your preceptor. You will also find it helpful to review your entries regularly in order to identify whether there are any patterns to the decisions you make that have resulted in unexpected outcomes: this may enable you to identify a knowledge deficit or an area for personal development. You may like to identify your decisions by type, as set out in Table 15.1.

Chapter summary

Decision-making is a skill which is developed and refined through experience. As you gain more experience you will find that your confidence in your ability to make decisions will increase. Increased confidence will allow you to involve patients more in the decision-making process, which will enhance their own self-esteem and locus of control. If at any time you are uncertain about a decision it is important to seek guidance as you will be accountable for all decisions you make.

Further reading

Benner, P (1984) *From Novice to Expert: Excellence and Power in Clinical Nursing Practice.* Menlo Park, CA: Addison Wesley.
This book provides excellent examples of how nurses make clinical judgements and the context within which they are made.

Standing, M (ed.) (2010) *Clinical Judgement and Decision-Making in Nursing and Interprofessional Healthcare.* Maidenhead: Open University Press.
This book covers the key knowledge, skills values and processes for clinical judgement and decision-making, with useful case studies showing how theory can be applied to practice.

Standing, M (2011) *Clinical Judgement and Decision Making for Nursing Students.* Exeter: Learning Matters.
Whilst aimed at students, this is an excellent introduction if you have not explored decision-making before.

Useful websites

There are some useful links to web resources on the Flying Start England website, which will provide you with evidence to support your decision-making. You will find these at:
www.flyingstartengland.nhs.uk/researchforpractice/judgements

There is a web activity on critical thinking on the Flying Start NHS website, which you will find at:
www.flyingstart.scot.nhs.uk/learning-programmes/research-for-practice/critical-appraisal.aspx

The Cochrane Library provides independent, high quality evidence to aid decision-making in healthcare:
www.thecochranelibrary.com

Chapter 16
Leadership and management development

Chapter aims

The aim of this chapter is to explore your role as a leader within a team. By the end of this chapter you will be able to:
- identify the skills required for managing and leading care;
- consider strategies you can use to lead a team effectively;
- identify your responsibilities with regard to delegation and appreciate the implications in delegating care activities;
- understand your role and responsibilities in supporting learners within the workplace.

Introduction

As a newly registered nurse you are likely to be one of the junior members of the team and may feel that leadership and management aren't relevant to you yet. However, within your team it is likely that there are members who are junior to you in terms of grading, as well as student nurses or student doctors and allied health professionals, all of whom will look to you for guidance. Depending on where you are working, you may have responsibility for a group of patients and work with a team of support workers and students to deliver their care; in this situation you will be required to use skills related to leadership and management. If you are working on a ward it is to be hoped that you will not be required to manage the whole ward during your preceptorship period, although unforeseen events such as significant staff sickness or adverse weather conditions preventing staff travelling to work could result in you being the most senior member of staff on duty, although it is likely that your employer would seek to provide appropriate support to you should this occur.

Leadership versus management

Leadership and management are two different concepts although they are often used interchangeably. A successful manager is likely to have effective leadership skills but you don't have to be a manager in order to be a leader. In both inpatient and community settings nurses undertake the role of team leader and while they may manage a case load they wouldn't be seen as managers. Sullivan and Garland (2010) define management and leadership as follows:

> *Management is about accomplishing the goals of the organisation through managing complexity so as to consistently ensure high standards, good practice and efficiency.*

> *Leadership is the intention to set direction, align efforts and motivate people to achieve results, which might involve managing change* (page 32).

Sullivan and Garland (2010) make the point that all nurses are managers from a practical perspective as they organise, plan and deliver care as well as directing the care to be delivered by others; also, all nurses are leaders as they influence how patient care is delivered and need to be able to respond to change. It is important, therefore, to start considering your strengths and areas for development in relation to your leadership and management skills.

Activity 16.1: Leadership and management

Management or leadership skills?

Reflect on your past experiences at work and think about individuals you have worked with who you believe had good management and/or leadership skills. What skills or attributes did they have that made you choose them? Is there a difference in the skill set they had? Which of these skills do you have and which do you think you need to develop?

There is a brief outline answer to this activity at the end of the chapter.

As a newly registered nurse you will require both leadership and management skills but not necessarily all the skills straight away. Key areas to focus on will be skills you have probably already acquired through your pre-registration programme or previous jobs that you have held but you probably feel that you need to gain more confidence in them within your new workplace. These skills are likely to be:

- effective communication and interpersonal skills including self-awareness;
- planning and organising skills;
- delegation skills;
- coaching and feedback skills.

Apart from the last set, each of the above skills will be needed whether you are working alone or in a team. The last set you are more likely to use when working with colleagues who have yet to acquire knowledge and/or skills in aspects of care in which you are competent and confident. They will therefore need both coaching to develop their competence and feedback from you on their progress. We will look at this later in this chapter.

Research summary: NHS Leadership Qualities Framework

The Hay Group were commissioned by the NHS to develop a leadership competency model which could be used for personal development as well as the support and development of leaders. The research involved reviewing over 20 leadership models and interviewing and consulting with more than 200 representatives of the NHS, Department of Health and patient representatives. The research resulted in a framework which identified 15 leadership qualities grouped under three headings:

- personal qualities: self-belief; self-awareness; self-management; drive for improvement; personal integrity;
- setting direction: broad scanning; intellectual flexibility; seizing the future; political astuteness; drive for results;
- delivering the service: leading change through people; holding to account; empowering others; collaborative working; effective and strategic influencing.

Each of the above qualities is broken down into a number of levels in the Framework, with examples of how each of the leadership qualities may be demonstrated at each of those levels. The Framework has been designed for leaders at all levels in the NHS but has applicability in any healthcare setting. The Framework and tools are available at **www. nhsleadershipqualities.nhs.uk/**

Leading a team

As discussed at the beginning of the chapter, depending on where you are working you may be expected to lead a team of colleagues such as healthcare support workers, students and possibly colleagues who are also newly registered. This leadership may be ongoing or ad hoc, depending on where you work and the skill mix within the team.

When you are asked to 'lead' a team it is essential that you spend some time at the start of the shift to identify the key priorities and agree who will undertake what tasks. This means that you need to know the capabilities of each member of your team and what they are permitted to do. Your role is likely to include all or some of the following:

- have knowledge of the condition and requirements of the patients/service users you are assigned to;
- delegate or assign specific responsibilities to each team member;
- co-ordinate patient activities delivered by the team;
- assist team members with care delivery;
- deliver direct care to patients/service users;
- liaise with other members of the multidisciplinary team;
- ensure effective communication within the team and external to the team;
- report to the charge nurse/manager any issues, concerns or challenges.

As you can see, this requires a range of skills but particularly important will be those of communication and delegation, and it is those we will look at next.

Delegation

As a registered nurse you will be working with other team members, carers and relatives and will need to make decisions as to who undertakes which activities when delivering care to patients and clients. In doing so you need to be very clear whether what you are doing is delegating activities or assigning them. They are very different and so have very different implications for you in relation to retaining or transferring accountability for the care undertaken.

Assignment happens when the activities assigned fall within that person's scope of practice and are set out in their role description.

Delegation is defined by the NMC (2008e) as *the transfer to a competent individual, the authority to perform a specific task in a specified situation that can be carried out in the absence of that nurse or midwife and without direct supervision.*

In the case of assignment, both responsibility and accountability are transferred to the person taking on the assigned activities, but when you delegate an activity you still retain accountability.

The NMC sets out your responsibilities with regard to delegation in the Code (NMC, 2008a) by stating that:

- *you must establish that anyone you delegate to is able to carry out your instructions;*
- *you must confirm that the outcome of any delegated task meets required standards;*
- *you must make sure that everyone you are responsible for is supervised and supported* (page 5).

Taking the above into account, you must consider a number of factors when making decisions about what activities are appropriate to delegate. For example:

- it must be in the best interest of the patient/client;
- the person delegated to must be competent to undertake the delegated activity (which will include having received the appropriate level of training for that activity);
- the person being delegated to must be clear as to their role and what is required of them;
- the level of supervision required must be agreed with clear lines of communication and feedback agreed regarding the activity to be undertaken.

Delegation and support workers

Changes in healthcare delivery have seen significant changes in the scope of professional practice in nursing. One of the consequences is that support workers are increasingly taking on what were once seen as nursing activities (Dimond, 2008; RCN, 2006). In most cases an employer will make decisions about what tasks support workers will undertake as part of their role. In this case the employer takes accountability for that decision but if you believe that the person to whom an activity has been delegated to is not competent to undertake it safely then you have a professional responsibility to intervene and let this be known (NMC, 2008e). On a day-to-day basis, however, you will need to use your professional judgement as to which tasks a support worker may also undertake. Remember that where a support worker is required to document the care given, it is your responsibility to ensure that they have documented appropriately.

Delegation and carers

Patients, service users and carers are increasingly being involved in care delivery as more care is delivered closer to or even at home. This is particularly true for carers or relatives of children who are caring for children at home. Although the carer/relative is not an employee, your responsibilities with regard to deciding what care activities can be delegated to them and to ensure that they receive the appropriate training remain the same and you will still be accountable for making that decision. The RCN identifies a list of procedures that can be delegated to carers who are caring for a child that is medically stable (RCN, 2008) and you will find that most community organisations will have a policy in place regarding the delegation of care to non-registrants which includes support workers and carers.

Delegation and students

The issue of delegation with regard to students is very different. They are not employees and the NMC (2008e) makes it clear that you must use your professional judgement in determining which activities a student can undertake and the level of supervision they will require when doing so. At all times the accountability remains with you; this relates to all activities that a student undertakes when working with you, either when directly or indirectly supervised by you.

The NMC's *Standards for Medicines Management* (NMC, 2008c) section 5 makes clear your responsibilities and accountability with regard to delegation in medicines management for students, support workers and carers. In each case you are accountable for ensuring that they are competent to carry out the task. With regard to students, you must always directly supervise them when they are administering medicines and if they sign the prescription chart you must countersign this.

Activity 16.2: Leadership and management

What activities may students not undertake?

Discuss what activities may not be delegated to student nurses with your manager, staff who are mentors to students, and the member of academic staff from your local university who is linked to your area (if there is one).

There is a brief outline answer to this activity at the end of the chapter.

> ## Case study: Bina makes assumptions about a student's capabilities
>
> *Bina has been asked to work with Tom, a second year student nurse, as his mentor has rung in sick. Bina hasn't worked with Tom before but has seen him around as he had been with them for a week and thought he appeared very confident and capable. She asks him if he knows how to take observations and he nods; so, thinking it will be a good experience for him, she asks him to care for a post-operative patient by taking his observations.*
>
> *Later in the shift Bina is completing her patients' notes and when she gets to the post-operative patient that Tom was caring for she finds that the patient has only had one set of observations completed on the chart. She checks the patient's wound site, which has been oozing considerably; the drains are full.*

In the case study Bina made a number of errors:

- she assumed Tom's air of confidence meant that he was competent;
- she assumed that he knew what the observation protocol was for a post-operative patient;
- she failed to check that he understood exactly what was required of him;
- she failed to supervise him to ensure that he was competent to undertake the task delegated.

Whilst Tom had a responsibility to inform Bina if he was unsure what was required of him, Bina at all times held accountability for his actions and would be required to answer for them.

Supporting learners in the workplace

Although a newly registered nurse, your learning has only just begun; you are on a lifelong journey of learning which will enrich your career and ensure that you meet the NMC's continuing professional development requirements. Alongside you there will be many others who are also continuing their learning journey, some of whom will look to you for support in meeting their learning needs. While you may feel that you have very little to offer as a newly registered nurse, anecdotal evidence from student nurses suggests that newly qualified nurses are particularly valued for the support they offer. Having so recently been students themselves, they have greater insight into a student's needs. Support workers undertaking National Vocational Qualifications (NVQs) or studying on a foundation degree may also look to you for support in helping them to develop their skills and knowledge.

Activity 16.3: Leadership and management

Role models
Reflect back on your experiences as a student nurse. Which mentors or nurses made a positive impression on you? What did they do or say that makes you remember them in a positive way? Which mentors or nurses had a negative impact on your practice experiences?

There is a brief outline answer to this activity at the end of the chapter.

By reflecting on your own experiences as a student, you will have identified the behaviours that 'good' mentors demonstrated that helped you to learn when in practice, and these should be the ones that you try to emulate, while making sure you avoid the ones you found unhelpful.

The NMC Code identifies your responsibilities with regard to supporting others, stating that *you must facilitate students and others to develop their competence* and that *you must be willing to share your skills and experience for the benefit of your colleagues* (NMC, 2008a). You cannot, however, act as a mentor during your preceptorship year as the NMC requires mentors to have been registered for at least one year before undertaking this role and to have completed an NMC-approved mentor preparation programme (NMC, 2008d). You can, however, facilitate student learning and provide feedback to them on their performance as well as acting as a role model to them. The NMC's *Standards to Support Learning and Assessment in Practice* (NMC, 2008d) has a four-stage developmental framework that enables you to plan your development from registrant to mentor and onwards if you wish to become a practice teacher or teacher. Table 16.1 outlines the outcomes relevant to a registered nurse or midwife who is not yet a qualified mentor or teacher, and so on stage one of the developmental framework.

Establishing effective working relationships	• work as a member of a multiprofessional team, contributing to team working • support those who are new to the team in integrating into the practice learning environment • act as a role model for safe and effective practice • develop effective working relationships based on mutual trust and respect
Facilitation of learning	• co-operate with those who have defined support roles contributing towards the provision of effective learning experiences • share their own knowledge and skills to enable others to learn in practice settings
Assessment and accountability	• work to the NMC Code for nurses and midwives in maintaining their own knowledge and proficiency for safe and effective practice • provide feedback to others in learning situations and to those who are supporting them so that learning is effectively assessed
Evaluation of learning	• contribute information related to those learning in practice, and about the nature of learning experiences, to enable those supporting students to make judgements on the quality of the learning environment
Create an environment for learning	• demonstrate a commitment to continuing professional development to enhance own knowledge and proficiency • provide peer support to others to facilitate their learning

continued opposite...

continued...

Context of practice	• whilst enhancing their own practice and proficiency, a registered nurse or midwife, act as a role model to others to enable them to learn their unique professional role
Evidence-based practice	• further develop their evidence base for practice to support their own professional development and to contribute to the development of others
Leadership	• use communication skills effectively to ensure that those in learning experiences understand their contributions and limitations to care delivery

Table 16.1: Standards for registrants to support learning and assessment in practice
Source: NMC (2008d)

There are eight domains in the standards with learning outcomes for each. The NMC expects the majority of registrants to meet the learning outcomes for stage one (NMC, 2008d). If you undertake an approved mentor preparation programme you will have met the learning outcomes for stage two. The expectations set out above are ones that you are probably meeting already. The skill that people usually find most challenging is giving feedback. Effective feedback skills are essential whether you are simply working with colleagues or supporting learners in the workplace.

Providing feedback

The provision of feedback to colleagues and the learners who you work with is important as it enables them to gain insight into their own performance; it helps them to have detailed information on what they are doing that is successful or requires improvement. Where the feedback is positive it can reinforce good practice, enhance a person's self-esteem and confidence and improve motivation (Clynes and Rafferty, 2008). Where improvement is needed, the information you give through feedback can provide them with the motivation to make the improvements required (Sullivan et al., 2009). If feedback is to be helpful it is important that you base it on evidence and also describe the impact of their actions in order that they can fully understand why their performance was effective or not. It is important to remember that feedback must always focus on performance, not on a person's character (Sharples, 2011). For instance, you might say they should ensure they make eye contact and smile when talking to a patient but not say they are unfriendly. If you have to provide feedback which includes areas for improvement, the 'feedback sandwich' can be a useful approach to use:

• give positive feedback on an aspect of performance;
• identify an area that requires improvement;
• give positive feedback on another aspect of performance.

The feedback sandwich enables the receiver to maintain self-esteem and so be more open to exploring how they can improve on their performance. As well as giving feedback you should also be seeking feedback on your own performance, not only from your preceptor but also from the members of the team you are working with, including students. Gaining feedback from multiple sources is called 360° feedback and it can be particularly helpful in gaining a wider perspective of your strengths and areas for improvement. It is also much easier for colleagues to accept feedback from you if you have accepted it in turn from them.

Chapter summary

This chapter has looked at leadership and management as it relates to you in your preceptorship year. Many of the skills required for effective management and leadership are also essential skills for effective nursing practice and so you should possess these already and you will develop the additional skills you require as you gain more experience. The skills of delegation and feedback may well be the most challenging initially, but will become easier with practice. Seeking feedback and reflecting on your own performance will enable you to further develop these skills.

Activities: brief outline answers

Activity 16.1: Management or leadership skills? (page 149)

It is likely that you have identified a list of skills that are the same for both effective managers and leaders. Jennings et al. (2007) found that there are a number of core skills shared by both, with the top four being:

- personal qualities;
- interpersonal skills;
- thinking skills;
- communication skills.

Skills that were seen as specific to leaders are their ability to communicate their vision of what nursing is and how to give high quality care and skills in developing people through mentoring and coaching. Leaders are also often seen to be enthusiastic and have the ability to inspire and motivate people and are determined to succeed and overcome barriers and challenges. In contrast, Jennings et al. (2007) found that competencies specific to managers were around human resource management and information management.

Activity 16.2: What activities may students not undertake? (page 152)

The list you come up with will depend on local policy and the policies of the university; however, it is likely to include:

- administration of medications via the intravenous route;
- administration of drugs under a patient group direction;
- escorting patients and clients on their own;
- using restraint techniques on patients/clients.

From an NMC perspective the only activities they give specific guidance on are in relation to medicines management. For all other activities it is the registered nurse's professional decision to determine whether a student is competent to undertake any activity but for some activities the student may be required to undertake specific training either locally or at the university before undertaking it (under supervision) in practice, e.g. restraint techniques, administration of blood and blood products, use of a blood glucose meter.

Activity 16.3: Role models (page 153)

While your answer to this activity will be very dependent on your personal experiences as a student, behaviours and attributes you may have identified are as follows:

- Positive experiences – made to feel welcome and part of the team, showed interest in your learning needs and gave feedback that was helpful. Myall et al. (2008) found students described positive experiences where mentors were *supportive, helpful, knowledgeable, experienced, enthusiastic about their role and committed to their students* (page 1837).
- Poor experiences of mentoring – these are likely to be the opposite to the above but are also likely to include mentors who were distant, unapproachable, intimidating or delegated the unwanted jobs to students (Gray and Smith, 2000).

Further reading

Elcock, K and Sharples, S (2010) *A Nurse's Survival Guide to Mentoring.* Edinburgh: Churchill Livingstone.
This book provides very practical guidance on supporting learners in practice.

Sullivan, E and Garland, G (2010) *Practical Leadership and Management.* Harlow, Essex: Pearson Education.
This book applies theory to practical situations with helpful case studies and tools you can use in the workplace.

Useful websites

To develop your confidence in giving feedback the section on feedback on the Flying Start England website provides some tips and activities that you may find useful. You will find these at: **www.flyingstartengland.nhs.uk/professional-development/feedback**

To get you started in thinking about your own workplace as a learning environment the Flying Start NHS website has an activity on this which you will find at: **www.flyingstart.scot.nhs.uk/learning-programmes/cpd/developing-others.aspx**

The Foundation of Nursing Leadership is a useful website that contains a range of resources including self-assessment tests, virtual seminars and a range of resources: **www.nursingleadership.org.uk/index.php**

Leadership Qualities Framework website provides a range of resources and advice for personal development advice around leadership: **www.nhsleadershipqualities.nhs.uk/**

Chapter 17
Developing an outcome approach to continuing professional development

Chapter aims

The aim of this chapter is to assist you in considering how you will plan your ongoing professional development. By the end of this chapter you will be able to:

- reflect on how the Knowledge and Skills Framework is relevant to you and your career;
- appreciate the importance of lifelong learning to your professional role;
- outline key changes and policy that will influence your future roles;
- develop a personal and professional development plan.

Where next?

The time of your preceptorship period will fly by as you get to grips with your new role and learn the many new skills required of you as a registered nurse. Most newly qualified nurses want to keep up the momentum of studying and are keen to undertake further study to progress their careers. Most employers will want you to concentrate on your preceptorship period first, but once you have achieved your first incremental point at around six months, it is time to start considering how you see your career progressing and what you need to do to achieve your aspirations. To start you thinking, look at Activity 17.1.

Activity 17.1: Evidence-based practice and research

Deciding your career pathway

Where do you see yourself in one year, in three years, and in five years?

What posts do you see yourself in? Do you know what knowledge, skills and qualifications you will require for these posts?

Take a look at the NHS jobs website, **www.jobs.nhs.uk**, and search for the posts you are aiming for and take a look at the person specifications. Each will identify the qualifications, experience, knowledge, skills and personal qualities/attitudes that are desirable and essential. What do you already have? What do you need to gain?

Make a note as this can feed into your personal development plan.

There is a brief outline answer to this activity at the end of the chapter.

From Activity 17.1 you will have identified areas in which you need to develop, so as to pursue your career pathway. Some of these areas can be achieved through further experience as a nurse; other areas will be achieved by undertaking informal or formal learning. Formal learning includes study days as well as short courses, such as specialist modules or a whole programme of study leading to an additional academic and/or professional qualification. Both formal and informal learning are important and both types of learning will contribute towards your continuing professional development.

Continuing professional development

Continuing Professional Development (CPD) is fundamental to the development of all health and social care practitioners, and is the mechanism through which high quality patient and client care is identified, maintained and developed, (RCN, 2007, page 2).

CPD is often talked about as something that is personal, as in 'my CPD'. While it is important to ensure that people are enabled to develop their roles and careers and you have a right to access CPD, CPD is much more than this. At the heart of CPD is the need to ensure that everyone in the healthcare workforce is equipped with the knowledge and skills not only to deliver high quality care for their clients and patients but also to ensure their safety. CPD is a requirement of both the NMC and the Knowledge and Skills Framework and therefore not something you can choose to do or not do. CPD is essential but sometimes there is confusion as to what activities you should undertake that can be counted towards your CPD.

CPD does not include the time you spend attending statutory or mandatory study days or sessions. Whilst these are important they are not tailored to your specific personal and professional development and are often generic to a range of healthcare workers. The NMC has set clear standards relating to CPD for nurses and midwives called the Prep standards (NMC, 2008b). Prep stands for post-registration education and practice and these standards can be downloaded from the NMC website, **www.nmc-uk.org**.

The NMC and Prep

When you first registered with the NMC you had to pay a fee and this will be an ongoing annual requirement as long as you wish to practise as a nurse. However, every third year you will be required to pay a renewal of registration fee *and* complete a notification of practice (NOP) form. In signing the NOP form you will be confirming to the NMC that you are of good health and good character and that you have met the NMC's Prep requirements (NMC, 2008b).

The NMC Prep requirements

There are two separate Prep standards that you are required to meet in order to maintain your registration, and these are set out in Table 17.1.

The Prep (practice) standard	You must have worked in some capacity by virtue of your nursing or midwifery qualification during the previous three years for a minimum of 450 hours, or have successfully undertaken an approved return to practice course within the last three years.
The Prep (continuing professional development) standard	You must have undertaken and recorded your continuing professional development (CPD) over the three years prior to the renewal of your registration… and you must have declared on your NOP form that you have met this requirement when you renew your registration.

Table 17.1: The NMC Prep standards
Source: NMC (2008b, page 6)

The NMC Prep (CPD) standard further specifies that you must:

- have undertaken 35 hours of learning activities over the last three years prior to the renewal of your registration;
- have recorded these 35 hours of learning activities in your professional profile.

The NMC does not detail specifically what the learning activities should be, but they do say that:

- *it doesn't have to cost you any money;*
- *there is no such thing as an approved Prep (CPD) learning activity;*
- *you don't need to collect points or certificates of attendance;*
- *there is no approved format for the personal professional profile;*
- *it must be relevant to the work you are doing or plan to do in the near future;*
- *it must help you to provide the highest possible standards of practice and care* (NMC, 2008b, page 12).

Examples of possible learning activities that the NMC suggests are:

- observing and learning a new skill;
- attending a seminar, teaching session or study day;
- completing a course either in-house or at an educational institution;

- reviewing published research underpinning an area of your practice to inform future practice;
- shadowing another member of staff;
- reading relevant reports/key papers published by journals/the Department of Health or other key organisations;
- networking with colleagues through specialist interest groups, formal or informal networks.

In each case whilst any of the above activities may be interesting or valuable, it is important that the ones you select are related to your work and you need to be able to demonstrate to the NMC that you have learnt from them. To do this you need to write a short reflection on this activity starting with 'The way in which this learning has influenced my work is…'. The NMC wants you to demonstrate what it is that you have learnt by undertaking this activity and how this will influence or has influenced the way you will work in the future. Simply reading an article or attending a study day is not enough; you need to identify what impact these activities have had on the way you practise as a nurse (see Case study 17.1).

Case study: Jaya undertakes research

Jaya has been caring for a patient who has had a permanent colostomy formed. She knows very little about the different types of colostomy bags and accessories available. She therefore looks up information on the Colostomy Association website, decides to register with them and is then able to download some of the factsheets and guidance sheets for nurses. She also arranges to spend half a day with the stoma nurse specialist at the hospital. Jaya then writes up a reflection for her professional profile, describing what she has learnt about colostomy bags and accessories and how this will change the way that she supports future patients who have a colostomy.

Activity 17.2: Critical thinking

Planning your profile

The NMC Prep standards outline the key headings you can use for your profile. Look at a copy of the Standards on the NMC website, **www.nmc-uk.org**, and use these headings to start your own profile. If you have access to a computer you can record this electronically – it doesn't have to be on paper, although you may want to keep any certificates of attendance together in a folder.

There is no outline answer to this activity as it is based on your own profile.

Chief Nursing Officer career pathway

In 2007 the Department of Health (DH) consulted on a post-registration framework for nursing careers which led to the development of a graphic representation of a pathway-based model which showed how nurses could progress their career either up through a speciality and/or across specialities following their preceptorship period. It recognises that nursing is no longer primarily based in a hospital but can take place in a wide range of settings including the community, people's homes, the workplace and the independent sector to name but a few. Key to this career pathway is the need for CPD to enable you to acquire the relevant skills and knowledge to progress through your chosen pathway. The diagrammatic representation is available on the Chief Nursing Officer's (CNO's) website at **www.dh.gov.uk/prod_consum_dh/groups/ dh_digitalassets/documents/digitalasset/dh_108369.pdf** and is summarised below.

There are five career pathways linked to patient pathways:

- family and public health;
- first contact, access and urgent care;
- supporting long term care;
- acute and critical care;
- mental health and psychosocial care.

Within each pathway you may choose to follow a career within one of these areas:

- clinical;
- management;
- education;
- research;

or you may move between them. For example, you may start out working as a nurse caring for clients with long term conditions, study for a teaching qualification and then become a Lecturer or Practice Educator teaching long term conditions.

Activity 17.3: Critical thinking

The CNO's careers pathway and you

Take a look at the CNO's diagram showing the different careers pathways for nurses: **www.dh.gov.uk/prod_consum_dh/groups/dh_digitalassets/documents/ digitalasset/dh_108369.pdf**. Now go back to your answers in Activity 17.1. Do your career plans fit with a specific pathway on the diagram? Would you change your answers to Activity 17.1 in any way having looked at the diagram?

There is no outline answer to this activity as it is based on your own profile.

Impact of the move to an all-graduate profession

Currently universities can provide pre-registration nursing programmes at diploma or degree level. However, following the publication of the NMC's new *Standards for Pre-registration Nursing Education* in 2010 all universities will be required to have moved to degree-only programmes by September 2013. Many qualified nurses are concerned about this change, with some worried that they will be viewed as less able if they do not have a degree. This is not the case.

First and foremost it is important to emphasise that the NMC differentiates between academic qualifications and professional qualifications. For example, three nurses could be studying to become a registered nurse and each exit with different academic qualifications: a diploma, a degree or a postgraduate diploma. However, each of them will have met the same professional requirements set by the NMC to register as a nurse and all of them will be recorded on part one of the NMC register as a registered nurse. Their academic level is not recorded.

If you already have a degree or postgraduate qualification in nursing the implications of this change will not immediately impact on you. However, if you qualified with a diploma or advanced diploma you may wish to consider how you can gain the extra academic credits you require to top up to a degree.

Why do I need a degree?

First, let's be absolutely clear. The NMC does not require you to have a degree if you are a registered nurse. However, there are two reasons why you should consider topping up your qualification to a degree if you do not already hold one.

Firstly, a degree will be required for your own career progression. If you aspire to more senior posts they are likely to require a degree or even a postgraduate qualification. The CNO's *Nursing Career Framework* (Department of Health, 2009) suggests that in the future senior posts such as ward managers, sisters, charge nurses, district nurses, clinical nurse specialists and community team leaders will either hold or be studying for a postgraduate diploma or master's degree and we will be seeing more senior posts studying for or holding a PhD!

Secondly, over the next few years you will find that more and more students that you come in contact with will be studying at degree level (with all students studying at degree level from 2013). While the NMC does not require you to hold the same academic qualification as the student you are mentoring you will find that topping up your qualification to a degree will help you develop greater skills of critical analysis, an enhanced understanding of research and evidence-based practice and greater confidence in the knowledge underpinning your practice which will in turn provide you with greater confidence in mentoring students.

If you choose not to top up to a degree you will still be required to demonstrate to the NMC when you renew your registration every three years that you have met their requirements for CPD, which does not have to result in academic credits or awards (NMC, 2008b) but may contribute to a degree or higher degree.

The annual appraisal and development of personal development reviews

An annual appraisal is essential if you are to effectively plan your personal and professional development. All healthcare organisations, no matter how small or large, should have an appraisal system in place. If you are working in the NHS and your employer has implemented the Agenda for Change Agreement (AfC) (2004a) and the NHS Knowledge and Skills Framework

(2004b) development tool, they are required to ensure that all staff receive an annual personal development review (PDR). The review will use your KSF post outline as the basis for the discussion that takes place. If you are not employed under AfC your employer should have an appraisal policy in place describing the process that should take place which you will need to access and follow.

Whilst your appraisal takes place on an annual basis you should be preparing for it throughout the year, especially if you are employed under AfC as you will be required to have collected evidence which demonstrates how your work compares to the relevant dimensions, levels and indicators in your KSF outline. Some NHS organisations use e-KSF, which is a web-based tool that enables staff to update and maintain their development review records online. The benefit of the online tool is that you can add your evidence as you collect it and continue to access your reviews if you move between NHS organisations. If you don't have access to e-KSF you will need to develop your own KSF portfolio.

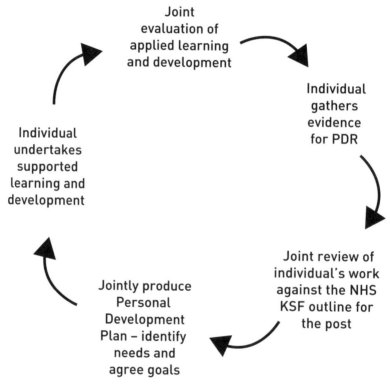

Figure 17.1: The development review cycle (adapted from Department of Health, 2004b)

The purpose of the development review is to look at:

- the duties and responsibilities of the individual's post and current agreed objectives;
- the application of knowledge and skills in the workplace;
- the consequent development needs of the individual.

Reviewers need to have regular informal discussions with the individual throughout the year, providing constructive feedback on their work and related development. All staff must have personal development plans in place that act as a foundation for these reviews. Development plans must relate to service need as well as the individual's aspirations for career development.

Chapter summary

Having registered as a nurse you are now committed to lifelong learning. As long as you wish to remain on the NMC register you will be required to demonstrate that you meet the NMC's requirements set out in their Prep standards. You will need to demonstrate clearly the outcomes of any CPD activities you have undertaken and record these in your professional profile. These outcomes must be relevant to your current area (or near future area) of practice.

Activities: brief outline answer

Activity 17.1: Deciding your career pathway (page 159)

The answers you gave to this activity will be personal to you. However, it is likely that you will have identified the need for any or all of the following:

- a minimum number of years of post-registration experience;
- a degree/masters degree;
- a mentorship qualification;
- completion of modules or a course related to the area of practice;
- teamwork/leadership/management skills.

Further reading

Nursing and Midwifery Council (2008) *The Prep Handbook*. London: NMC. Available at **www.nmc-uk.org**

Royal College of Nursing (2006) *Discussing and Preparing Evidence at your First Personal Development Review: Guidance for RCN Members on the NHS Knowledge and Skills Framework*. RCN: London. Available at **www.rcn.org.uk**

Useful websites

To develop your skills in managing your own continuing professional development, there are a series of continuing development activities on the Flying Start England website that you may find useful to complete. You will find the details of this activity at: **www.flyingstartengland.nhs.uk/professional-development/cpd**

NHS Jobs is an online recruitment service advertising thousands of jobs. It provides lots of advice on how to apply for a job as well as preparing for your interview. See **www.jobs.nhs.uk**

NHS Employers provides a wealth of information about working in the NHS. See **www.nhsemployers.org**

Skills for Health provides a range of information, resources and guides you can use to plan your professional development, including information regarding careers in the independent sector. See **www.skillsforhealth.org.uk**

e-KSF is a web-based toolkit for implementing the KSF (**www.e-ksfnow.org/**) and provides some useful examples of the review process.

References

Agenda for Change Project Team (2004) *The NHS Knowledge and Skills Framework (NHS KSF) and the Development Review Process.* London: Department of Health Publications.

Almost, J (2006) Conflict within nursing work environments: a concept analysis. *Journal of Advanced Nursing*, 53 (4): 444–53.

Anders, H, Douglas, D and Harrigan, R (1995) Competencies of new registered nurses – a survey of deans and health care agencies in the state of Hawaii. *Nursing Connections*, 8 (3): 5–16.

Atkins, S and Murphy, K (1995) Reflective practice. *Nursing Standard*, 9 (45): 31–35.

Atwal, A and Caldwell, K (2005) Do all health and social care professionals interact equally: a study of interactions in multidisciplinary teams in the United Kingdom. *Scandinavian Journal of Caring Science*, 19: 268–73.

Atwal, A and Caldwell, K (2006) Nurses' perceptions of multidisciplinary team work in acute health-care. *International Journal of Nursing Practice*, 12: 359–65.

Bach, S and Grant, A (2009) *Communication and Interpersonal Skills for Nurses.* Exeter: Learning Matters.

Balzer-Riley, J (2000) *Communication in Nursing*, 4th edn. St Louis: Mosby.

Bandura, A (1977) Self-efficacy: toward a unifying theory of behavioural change. *Psychological Review*, 84 (2): 191–215.

Bandura, A and MacDonald, F (1963) Influence of social reinforcement and the behaviour of models in shaping children's moral judgements. *Journal of Abnormal and Social Psychology*, 67: 274–81.

Banning, M (2005) Conceptions of evidence, evidenced based medicine, evidenced based practice and their use in nursing: independent nurse prescribers' views. *Journal of Clinical Nursing*, 14: 411–17.

Banning, M (2007) A review of clinical decision making: models and current research. *Journal of Clinical Nursing*, 17 (2): 187–95.

Baxter, C (2001) *Managing Diversity & Inequality in Health Care.* London: Bailliere Tindall.

Begley, C and Brady, A (2002) Irish diploma in nursing students' first clinical allocation: the views of nurse managers. *Journal of Nursing Management*, 10: 339–47.

Belbin, RM (2010) *Management Teams: Why They Succeed or Fail*, 3rd edn. Oxford: Butterworth-Heinemann.

Benjamin, D (2001) Reducing medication errors and increasing patient safety through better communication. *Focus on Patient Safety*, 4 (4): 6,8.

Benner P (1984) *From Novice to Expert: Excellence and Power in Clinical Nursing Practice.* Menlo Park, CA: Addison Wesley.

Benner, P and Tanner, C (1987) Clinical judgment: How expert nurses use intuition. *American Journal of Nursing*, 87: 23–31.

Bircumshaw, D (1990) the utilisation of research findings in clinical practice. *Journal of Advanced Nursing*, 15: 1272–80.

Blakemore, S (2009) Good equality policies can save each trust £8.3 million a year. *Nursing Standard*, 23(35): 9.

Borrill, C, West, M, Dawson, J, Shapiro, D, Rees, A, Richards, A, Garrod, S, Carletta, J and Carter, A (2002) *Team Working and Effectiveness in Healthcare: Findings from the Healthcare Team Effectiveness Project.* Birmingham: Aston Centre for Health Service Organisation Research, Aston University.

Boud, D and Walker, D (1993) Barriers to reflection on experience, in Boud, D, Cohen, R and Walker, D (eds) *Using Experience for Learning.* Buckingham: The Society for Research into Higher Education and Open University Press.

Boud, D, Keogh, R and Walker, D (1985) *Reflection: Turning Experience into Learning.* London: Kogan Page.

Brookfield, S (1994) Adult learning: an overview, in Tuinjman, A (ed.) *International Encyclopaedia of Education.* Oxford: Pergamon Press.

Cahill, H (1996) A qualitative analysis of student nurses' experiences of mentorship. *Journal of Advanced Nursing*, 24: 791–99.

Cantor, J (1995) *Experiential Learning in Higher Education.* Washington: The George Washington University.

Chitty, K (2005) *Professional Nursing: Concepts & Challenges.* Missouri: Elsevier Saunders.

Cleary, M and Freeman, A (2005) Email etiquette: Guidelines for mental health nurses. *International Journal of Mental Health nursing*, 14: 62–65.

Clynes, M and Rafferty, S (2008) Feedback: An essential element of student learning in clinical practice. *Nurse Education in Practice*, 8 (6): 405–11.

Colin-Thome, D (2009) *Mid Staffordshire NHS Foundation Trust: A review of lessons learnt for commissioners and performance managers following the Healthcare Commission investigation.* Available at: www.midstaffsinquiry.com, last accessed 12 May 2011.

Cook, M (2008) Care management, in Spouse J, Cook, M and Cox, C (eds) *Common Foundation Studies in Nursing*, 4th edn. Edinburgh: Churchill Livingstone.

Cooke, H and Philpin, S (2008) *Sociology in Nursing and Healthcare.* Edinburgh: Churchill Livingstone.

Curtin, L (1979) The nurse as advocate: a philosophical foundation for nursing. *Advances in Nursing Science*, 1 (3): 1–10.

Cutcliffe, JT and Stevenson, C (2008) Never the twain? Reconciling national suicide prevention strategies with the practice educational, and policy needs of mental health nurses (Part two). *International Journal of Mental Health Nursing*, 17: 351–62.

Davis, C (2007) Keeping the peace. *Nursing Standard*, 22 (12): 18–19.

Dennison, B and Kirk, R (1990) *Do, Review, Learn, Apply: A Simple Guide to Experiential Learning.* Oxford: Blackwell Education.

Department of Health (2000) *The NHS Plan. A Plan for Change. A Plan for Reform.* London: Department of Health.

Department of Health (2001a) *Working Together – Learning Together: A Framework for Lifelong Learning for the NHS.* London: Department of Health.

Department of Health (2001b) *Learning from Bristol: The Report of the Public Inquiry into Children's Heart Surgery at the Bristol Royal Infirmary.* London: Stationery Office, Department of Health.

Department of Health (2002) *Extension of Independent Nurse Prescribing.* London: Department of Health.

Department of Health (2004a) *Agenda for Change Final Agreement.* London: Department of Health, available at www.dh.gov.uk/en/Publicationsandstatistics/Publications/PublicationsPolicyAndGuidance/DH_4095943, last accessed 27 March 2011.

Department of Health (2004b) *NHS Knowledge and Skills Framework and the Development Review Process.* London: Department of Health, available at www.dh.gov.uk/en/Publicationsandstatistics/Publications/PublicationsPolicyAndGuidance/DH_4090843, last accessed 27 March 2011.

Department of Health (2008a) *A High Quality Workforce. NHS Next Stage Review.* London: Department of Health.

Department of Health (2008b) *High Quality Care for All – NHS Next Stage Review Final Report.* London: Department of Health.

Department of Health (2009) *Nursing Career Framework*, available at www.dh.gov.uk/en/Aboutus/Chiefprofessionalofficers/Chiefnursingofficer/DH_108368, last accessed 27 March 2011.

Department of Health (2010a) *Preceptorship Framework for Newly Registered Nurses, Midwives and Allied Health Professionals*, available at www.dh.gov.uk/prod_consum_dh/groups/dh_digitalassets/@dh/@en/@abous/documents/digitalasset/dh_114116.pdf, last accessed 27 March 2011.

Department of Health (2010b) *NHS Constitution*, available at http://www.nhs.uk/choiceintheNHS/Rightsandpledges/NHSConstitution/Pages/Overview.aspx, last accessed 27 March 2011.

Department of Health (2010c) *Equity and Excellence: Liberating the NHS.* Norwich: The Stationery Office.

Dewey, J (1933) *How we Think: A Restatement of the Relation of Reflective Thinking to the Educative Process.* New York: Health and Co.

Dimond, B (2008) *Legal Aspects of Nursing*, 5th edn. Harlow: Pearson Education.

Duchscher, J (2001) Out in the real world: newly graduated nurses in acute care speak out. *Journal of Nursing Administration*, 31: 426–29.

Eby, M (2000) *The Challenges of Being Accountable. Critical Practice in Health and Social Care* (eds A Brechin, H Brown and M Eby). London: Sage.

Elcock, K (1997) Reflections on being therapeutic and reflection. *Nursing in Critical Care*, 2 (3): 138–43.

Elcock, K (2008) Developing and sustaining the advanced practitioner role, in Neno, R and Price, D (eds) *The Handbook for Advanced Primary Care Nurses.* Maidenhead: Open University Press.

Equality Act (2010). London: HMSO, available at www.equalities.gov.uk/equality_act_2010.aspx, last accessed 27 March 2011.

Eraut, M (2006) Editorial. *Learning in Health and Social Care*, 5 (3): 111–18.

Foley, B, Minick, P and Kee, C (2000) Nursing advocacy during military operation. *Western Journal of Nursing Research*, 22: 492–507.

Fowler, J (1998) *The Handbook of Clinical Supervision – Your Questions Answered.* Salisbury: Quay Books.

Foy, C and Timmins, F (2004) Improving communication in day surgery settings. *Nursing Standard*, 19 (7): 37–42.

Frances, R (2010) *The Mid Staffordshire NHS Foundation Trust Inquiry.* London: HMSO.

Frith, L (1999) Clinical Risk Modification and Ethics, in Wilson, J and Tingle, J (eds) *Clinical Risk Modification.* Edinburgh: Butterworth Heinemann.

Ghaye, T and Lillyman, S (eds) (2000) *Effective Clinical Supervision: the Role of Reflection.* Wiltshire: Quay Books.

Gibbons, M (1993) Listening to the lived experience of loss. *Paediatric Nursing*, 6: 597–99.

Gibbs, G (1988) *Learning by Doing: A Guide to Teaching and Learning Methods.* Oxford: Further Education Unit, Oxford Polytechnic.

Glover, P (2000) 'Feedback. I listened, reflected and utilized': Third year nursing students' perceptions and use of feedback in the clinical setting. *International Journal of Nursing Practice*, 6: 247–52.

Godinez, G, Schweiger, J, Gruver, J and Ryan, P (1999) Role transition from graduate nurse to staff nurse: A qualitative analysis. *Journal of Staff Development*, 15 (3): 97–110.

Gray, MA and Smith, LN (2000) The qualities of an effective mentor from the student nurse's perspective: Findings from a longitudinal qualitative study. *Journal of Advanced Nursing*, 32(6): 1542–49.

Greenberg, L (2007) Emotion in the therapeutic relationship in emotion–focused therapy, in Gilbert, P and Leahy, R (eds) *The Therapeutic Relationship in the Cognitive Behavioural Psychotherapies.* Hove: Routledge.

Hall, C and Ritchie, D (2009) *What is Nursing? Exploring Theory and Practice.* Exeter: Learning Matters.

Hammond, KR (1996) *Human Judgement and Social Policy: Irreducible uncertainty, inevitable error, unavoidable injustice.* New York: Oxford University Press.

Hanks, R (2010) Development and testing of an instrument to measure protective nursing advocacy. *Nursing Ethics*, 17 (2): 255–67.

Harmer, S (2005) Evidenced based practice, in Harmer, S and Collinson, G (eds) *Achieving Evidenced based Practice*, 2nd edn. London: Balliere Tindall.

Healthcare Commission (2006) *Investigation into outbreaks of Clostridium difficile at Stoke Mandeville Hospital, Buckinghamshire Hospitals NHS Trust July 2006.* London: Commission for Healthcare Audit and Inspection.

Healthcare Commission (2007) *Investigation into outbreaks of Clostridium difficile at Maidstone and Tunbridge Wells NHS Trust.* London: Commission for Healthcare Audit and Inspection.

Healthcare Commission (2009) *Investigation into Mid Staffordshire NHS Foundation Trust.* London: Commission for Healthcare Audit and Inspection.

Health Education Authority (1999) *Risk Assessment at Work: Practical Examples in the NHS.* London: Health Education Authority.

Hek, G and Shaw, A (2006) The contribution of research knowledge and skills to practice: an exploration of the views and experiences of newly qualified nurses. *Journal of Research in Nursing*, 11 (6): 473–82.

Hendrick, J (2000) *Law and Ethics in Nursing and Healthcare.* Cheltenham: Stanley Thornes.

Hendrick, J (2010) *Law and Ethics in Children's Nursing.* Oxford: Wiley-Blackwell.

Higgens, G, Spencer, RL and Kane, R (2010) A systematic review of the experiences and perceptions of the newly qualified nurse in the United Kingdom. *Nurse Education Today*, 30: 499–508.

Hobbs, J and Green, S (2003) Development of a preceptorship programme. *British Journal of Midwifery*, 11 (6): 372–75.

Hole, J (2009) *The Newly Qualified Nurses' Survival Guide.* Oxford: Radcliffe Publishing.

Holland, K, Roxburgh, M, Johnson, M, Topping, K, Watson, R, Lauder, W and Porter, M (2010) Fitness for practice in nursing and midwifery education in Scotland, United Kingdom. *Journal of Clinical Nursing*, 19: 461–69.

Holmes-Bonney, K (2010) Managing complaints in health and social care. *Nursing Management*, 17(1): 12–15.

Honey, P and Mumford, A (1992) *The Manual of Learning Styles.* Maidenhead: Peter Honey Publications.

Hughes, J and Pakieser, R (1999) Factors that impact on nurses use of electronic mail. *Computers in Nursing*, 17: 251–58.

Humphris, D (2005) Types of evidence, in Harmer, S and Collinson, G (eds) *Achieving Evidenced based Practice*, 2nd edn. London: Balliere Tindall.

INSA bulletin (2010) Whose job is it anyway? The nurse's role in advocacy and accountability. *Indiana State Nurse Association*, February/March/April.

Ipsos MORI (2010) *Violence against frontline NHS staff – Research for COI on behalf of the NHS Security Management Service*, available at www.nhsbsa.nhs.uk/Documents/SecurityManagement/NHS_SMS_Workplace_Safety_Report_FINAL_MERGED.pdf, last accessed 27 March 2011.

Jack, K and Smith, A (2007) Promoting self-awareness in nurses to improve nursing practice. *Nursing Standard*, 21 (32): 47–52.

Jarrett, N and Payne, S (1995) A selective review of the literature on nurse patient communication: Has the patient's contribution been neglected? *Journal of Advanced Nursing*, 22 (1): 72–78.

Jarvis, P, Holford, J and Griffin, C (1998) *The Theory and Practice of Learning*. London: Kogan Page.

Johns, C (2004) *Becoming a Reflective Practitioner*, 2nd edn. Oxford: Blackwell Publishing.

Jomeen, J, Wray, J, Stimpson, A, Whitfield, C and McCulloch, A (2008) *Review of Student Guidance for Professional Behaviour.* Hull: University of Hull.

Joyce, L (2005) Applying the evidence, in Harmer, S and Collinson, G (eds) *Achieving Evidenced based Practice*, 2nd edn. London: Balliere Tindall.

Klardie, K, Johnson, J, McNaughton, M and Meyers, W (2004) Integrating the principles of evidenced based practice into clinical practice. *Journal of the American Academy of Nurse Practitioners*, 16 (3): 98–105.

Knowles, M, Holton, E and Swanson, R (1998) *The Adult Learner*, 5th edn. Houston: Gulf.

Kolb, D (1984) *Experiential Learning: Experience as the Source of Learning and Development*. Englewood Cliffs, NJ: Prentice Hall.

Kramer, M (1974) *Reality Shock: Why Nurses Leave Nursing*. St Louis: Mosby.

Laming Report (2003) *The Victoria Climbé Inquiry. Report of an inquiry by Lord Laming*. London: HMSO.

Learner, S. (2006) Fears for literacy and numeracy as new nurses fail basic tests. *Nursing Standard*, 20 (49): 10.

Leathard, A (2003) *Interprofessional Collaboration from Policy to Practice in Health and Social Care*. Hove: Brunner-Routledge.

Lee, R (2007) Responsibility, liability and scarce resources, in Tingle, J and Cribb, A (eds) *Nursing Law and Ethics*, 3rd edn. Oxford: Blackwell.

Légaré, F, Ratté, S, Stacey, D, Kryworuchko, J, Gravel, K, Graham, ID and Turcotte, S (2010) *Interventions for improving the adoption of shared decision making by healthcare professionals (Review): Cochrane Database of Systematic Reviews* 2010, Issue 5. Art. No.: CD006732. DOI: 10.1002/14651858.CD006732.pub2.

Leners, D, Roehrs, C and Piccone, A (2005) Tracking the Development of Professional Values in Undergraduate Nursing Students. *Journal of Nursing Education*, 45 (12): 504–11.

Lewis, C (2006) *Clinical Negligence*. London: Tottel.

Light, G, Cox, R and Calkins, S (2009) *Learning and Teaching in Higher Education: The Reflective Professional*, 2nd edn. London: Sage.

Llewellyn, P and Northway, R (2010) An investigation into the advocacy role of the learning disability nurse. *Journal of Research in Nursing*, 12: 147–60.

LoBiondo-Wood, G (1990) *Nursing Research: Methods, Critical Appraisal and Utilisation*, 2nd edn. St Louis: Mosby.

Luft, J (1969) *Of Human Interaction*. Palo Alto, CA: National Press.

Maben, J, Latter, S and Macleod Clark, J (2007) The sustainability of ideals, values and the nursing mandate: evidence from a longitudinal qualitative study. *Nursing Inquiry*, 44 (2): 99–113.

Makoul, G and Clayman, ML (2006) An integrative model of shared decision making in medical encounters. *Patient Education and Counselling*, 60 (3): 301–12.

Mallik, M (1997) Advocacy in nursing – a review of the literature. *Journal of Advanced Nursing*, 25 (1): 130–38.

Markanday, L (1997) *Day Surgery for Nurses*. London: Whurr.

Maughan, B and Conduit, A (1999) Complaints: the patients perspective, in Wilson, J and Tingle, J (eds) *Clinical Risk Modification*. Edinburgh: Butterworth Heinmann.

McCabe, C and Timmins, F (2006) *Communication Skills for Nursing Practice*. Basingstoke: Palgrave Macmillan.

Mitchell, M (1997) Patients' perceptions of pre-operative preparation for day surgery. *Journal of Advanced Nursing*, 26 (2): 356–63.

Mooney, M (2006) Facing registration: The expectations and the unexpected. *Nurse Education Today*, 27: 840–47.

Mottram, J and Pickens, S (2000) Clinical Audit: Watching the detectives. *Health Service Journal*. 110 (5689): 26–7.

Muir, N (2004) Clinical decision-making: theory and practice. *Nursing Standard*, 18 (36): 47–52.

Myall, M, Levett-Jones, T and Lathlean, J (2008) Mentorship in contemporary practice: the experiences of nursing students and practice mentors. *Journal of Clinical Nursing*, 17: 1834–42.

Nancarrow, S and Borthwick, A (2005) Dynamic professional boundaries in the healthcare workforce. *Sociology of Health and Illness*, 27 (7): 897–919s.

National Audit Office (NAO) (2003) *A Safer Place to Work – Protecting NHS Hospital and Ambulance Staff from Violence and Aggression*. London: NAO.

National Confidential Inquiry into Suicide and Homicide by People with Mental Illness (2006) *Avoidable Deaths: five year report of the national confidential inquiry into suicide and homicide by people with mental illness*. Manchester: University of Manchester.

National Patient Safety Agency (2009) *Review of Patient Safety for Children and Young People*: NPSA: London, www.npsa.nhs.uk.

National Steering Group for Decision Support Aids in Urology (2005) *Implementing Patient Decision Aids in Urology–Final Report*. Oxford: Picker Institute Europe.

Nelson-Jones, R (2006) *Human Relationship Skills: Coaching and Self-Coaching*, 4th edn. Hove, West Sussex: Routledge.

Newdick, C (2005) *Who Should we Treat?*, 2nd edn. Oxford: Oxford University Press.

NHS (2008) *SBAR*. Institute for Innovation and Improvement. Available from: www.institute.nhs.uk/quality_and_service_improvement_tools/quality_and_service_improvement_tools/sbar_-_situation_-_background_-_assessment_-_recommendation.html.

NHS Choices (2010) *Same-sex Accommodation*. Available from: www.nhs.uk/choiceintheNHS/Rightsandpledges/samesexaccommodation/Pages/Overview.aspx.

NHS East of England (2007) *General Practice Nursing Preceptorship and Assessment Booklet*. Cambridge: NHS East of England Deanery.

NHS Employers (2009) *Managing Diversity: Making it Core Business*. London: NHS Employers.

NHS Institute for Innovation and Improvement (2003) *NHS Leadership Qualities Framework: The Full Technical Research Paper*, available at www.nhsleadershipqualities.nhs.uk, last accessed 27 March 2011.

NHS Institute for Innovation and Improvement (2005) *NHS Leadership Qualities Framework*, available at www.nhsleadershipqualities.nhs.uk, last accessed 27 March 2011.

NHS Institute for Innovation and Improvement (2009) *High Impact Interventions for Nursing and Midwifery.* Warwick: NHS Institute for Innovation and Improvement.

NHSLA (2010) *Key Facts about our Work.* NHS Litigation Authority. Available from: www.nhsla.com/home. htm.

NHS Modernisation Agency (2004) *10 High Impact Changes for Service Improvement and Delivery: A Guide for NHS Leaders.* London: Department of Health.

NHS Staff Council (2010) *NHS Terms and Conditions of Service Handbook Amendment number 17 Pay Circular (AforC) 2/2010*, available at www.nhsemployers.org, last accessed 27 March 2011.

Norton, D (1988) *Remembered with Advantage, Research Efforts Gone By.* London: Royal Collage of Nursing.

NPSA (2008) *Briefing: Act on Reporting.* London: NHS Confederation Publication.

NPSA (2009) *Never Events Framework 2009/2010.* London: NHS Confederation Publication.

NPSA (2010) *Reducing Harm from Omitted and Delayed Medicines in Hospital.* London: NHS Confederation Publication.

Nursing and Midwifery Council (2004) *Standards of Proficiency for Pre-registration Nursing Education.* London: NMC, available from: www.nmc-uk.org.

Nursing and Midwifery Council (2006) *Preceptorship Guidelines*, NMC Circular 21/2006. London: NMC, available at www.nmc-uk.org, last accessed 27 March 2011.

Nursing and Midwifery Council (2008a) *The Code: Standards of Conduct, Performance and Ethics for Nurses and Midwives.* London: NMC, available from: www.nmc-uk.org.

Nursing and Midwifery Council (2008b) *The PREP Handbook.* London: NMC, available at www.nmc-uk. org, last accessed 27 March 2011.

Nursing and Midwifery Council (2008c) *Standards for Medicines Management.* London: NMC, available at www.nmc-uk.org, last accessed 27 March 2011.

Nursing and Midwifery Council (2008d) *Standards to Support Learning and Assessment in Practice. NMC Standards for Mentors, Practice Teachers and Teachers.* London: NMC, available at: www.nmc.-uk.org, last accessed 27 March 2011.

Nursing and Midwifery Council (2008e) *Advice on Delegation.* London: NMC, available at: www.mnc-uk. org, last accessed 27 March 2011.

Nursing and Midwifery Council (2009a) *Guidance on Professional Conduct for Nursing and Midwifery Students.* London: NMC, available at www.nmc-uk.org, last accessed 27 March 2011.

Nursing and Midwifery Council (2009b) *Fitness to Practice Annual Report*: 1 April 2008 to 31 March 2009. London: NMC, available at www.nmc-uk.org.

Nursing and Midwifery Council (2009c) *Accountability.* London: NMC, available at www.nmc-uk.org, last accessed 27 March 2011.

Nursing and Midwifery Council (2010a) *Standards for Pre-registration nursing Education.* London: NMC, available from: www.nmc-uk.org, last accessed 27 March 2011.

Nursing and Midwifery Council (2010b) *Record Keeping: Guidance for Nurses and Midwives.* London: NMC, available from: www.nmc-uk.org, last accessed 27 March 2011.

Nursing and Midwifery Council (2010c) *Raising and Escalating Concerns: Guidance for Nurses and Midwives.* London: NMC, available from: www.nmc-uk.org, last accessed 27 March 2011.

O'Connor, S, Pearce, J, Smith, R, Voegeli, D and Walton, P (2001) An evaluation of the clinical performance of newly qualified nurses: a competency based assessment. *Nurse Education Today*, 21 (7): 559–68.

O'Grady, L and Jadad, A (2010) Shifting from Shared to Collaborative Decision Making: A Change in Thinking and Doing. *Journal of Participatory Medicine*, 2: e13.

Olson, M (2009) The 'Millennials': First year in practice. *Nursing Outlook*, 57 (1): 10–17.

Packham, C (2010) *Violence at Work: Findings from the 2009/10 British Crime Survey.* London: Home Office.

Pajares, F (2002) Overview of social cognitive theory and of self-efficacy. Available from: www.emory.edu/EDUCATION/mfp/eff.html.

Parliamentary and Health Service Ombudsman (2010) *Listening and Learning: the Ombudsman's review of complaint handling by the NHS in England 2009-10.* London: The Stationery Office.

Parliamentary and Health Service Ombudsman (2011) *Care and Compassion? Report of the Health Service Ombudsman on ten investigations into NHS care of older people.* London: The Stationery Office.

Patient Opinion (2011) *In their Words. What Patients think about our NHS*, available at www.patientopinion.org.uk/resources/POreport2011.pdf, last accessed 27 March 2011.

Pattison, D, Parsons, D and Weatherhead, C (2000) Connecting reflective practice with clinical supervision, in Ghaye, T and Lillyman, S (eds) *Effective Clinical Supervision: the Role of Reflection.* Wiltshire: Quay Books.

Pearce, C. (2007) Ten steps to carrying out a SWOT analysis. *Nursing Management*, 14 (92): 25.

Poroch, D and McIntosh, W (1995) Barriers to assertive skills in nurses. *Australian and New Zealand Journal of Mental Health Nursing*, 4: 113–23.

Pugh, B (1992) Feedback in clinical teaching. *Nurse Educator*, 17 (1): 5–7.

Racia, D (2009) Effect of action-orientated communication training on nurses' communication self-efficacy. *Medsurg Nursing*, 18 (6): 343–60.

Rahim, MA (2010) *Managing Conflict in Organizations*, 4th edn. New Brunswick, New Jersey: Transaction Publishers.

Robb, R, Jarman, B, Suntharalingam, G, Higgens, C, Tennant, R and Elcock, K (2010) Using care bundles to reduce in-hospital mortality: quantitative survey. *British Medical Journal*, 340: c1234: 61–863.

Roberts, D (2009) Newly qualified nurses: Competence or confidence. *Nurse Education Today*, 29: 467–68.

Robinson, S and Griffiths, P (2009) *Scoping review Preceptorship for Newly Qualified Nurses: Impacts, Facilitators and Constraints.* London: King's College London National Nursing Research Unit.

Rosenberg, W and Donald, A (1995) Evidenced based medicine: an approach to clinical problem solving. *British Medical Journal*, 310: 1122–26.

Roxburgh, M, Lauder, W, Topping, K, Holland, K, Johnson, M and Watson, R (2010) Early findings from an evaluation of a post-registration staff development programme: The Flying Start NHS initiative in Scotland, UK. *Nurse Education in Practice*, 10: 76–81.

Royal College of Nursing (2006) *Discussing and Preparing Evidence at your First Personal Development Review: Guidance for RCN Members on the NHS Knowledge and Skills Framework.* London: RCN.

Royal College of Nursing (2007) *A Joint Statement on Continuing Professional Development for Health and Social Care Practitioners*, available at www.rcn.org.uk, last accessed 27 March 2011.

Royal College of Nursing (2008) *Managing Children with Health Care Needs: Delegation of Clinical Procedures, Training and Accountability Issues.* London: RCN.

Schoessler, M and Waldo, M (2006) The first 18 months practice: A developmental transitional model for the newly graduated nurse. *Journal for Nurses in Staff Development*, 22 (2): 47–52.

Schon, D (1983) *The Reflective Practitioner.* Aldershot: Avebury.

Schon, DA (1987) *Educating the Reflective Practitioner: Toward a New Design for Teaching and Learning in the Professions.* San Francisco: Jossey-Bass.

Scott, J, Ingram, J and Mackenzie, F (2010) The effectiveness of drug round tabards in reducing incidence of medication errors. *Nursing Times.* 106 (34): 13–15.

Sharples, K (2009) *Learning to Learn in Nursing Practice.* Exeter: Learning Matters.

Standing, M (2005) Perceptions of Clinical Decision-making on a Developmental Journey from Student to Staff Nurse, PhD Thesis, Canterbury, University of Kent.

Sharples, K (2011) Giving Feedback, in Elcock K and Sharples K (eds) *A Nurse's Survival Guide to Mentoring.* Edinburgh: Churchill Livingston.

Standing, M (2008) Clinical judgement and decision-making in nursing – nine modes of practice in a revised cognitive continuum. *Journal of Advanced Nursing*, 62(1): 124–34.

Standing, M (ed.) (2010) *Clinical Judgement and Decision-Making in Nursing and Interprofessional Healthcare.* Maidenhead: Open University Press.

Sullivan, E and Garland, G (2010) *Practical Leadership and Management.* Harlow, Essex: Pearson Education.

Sutherland, P and Crowther, J (eds) (2006) *Lifelong Learning.* London: Routledge.

Taris, T and Feij, J (2004) Learning and strain in newcomers: a three-wave study on the effects of job demands and job control. *Journal of Psychology*, 138: 543–63.

The Lord Lamming (2009) *The Protection of Children in England: A Progress Report.* London: The Stationery Office.

Thomas, KW and Kilmann, RH (1974) *Thomas–Kilmann Conflict Mode Instrument.* Mountain View, CA: Xicom.

Thompson, C and Dowding, D (eds) (2002) *Clinical Decision Making and Judgement in Nursing.* Edinburgh: Churchill Livingstone.

Thompson, C and Dowding, D (eds) (2009) *Essential Decision Making and Clinical Judgement for Nurses.* Edinburgh: Churchill Livingstone.

Thompson, C, McCaughan, D, Cullum, N, Sheldon, TA, Thompson, DR and Mulhall, A (2001) *Nurses' Use of Research Information in Clinical Decision making: A Descriptive and Analytical Study.* York: University of York.

Thompson, IE, Melia, KM and Boyd, KM (2006) *Nursing Ethics*, 5th ed. Edinburgh: Churchill Livingstone.

Timmins, F (2008) *Making Sense of Portfolios: A Guide for Nursing Students.* Maidenhead: Open University Press.

United Kingdom Central Council for Nursing, Midwifery and Health Visiting (1986) *Project 2000: a New Preparation for Practice.* London: UKCC.

United Kingdom Central Council for Nursing, Midwifery and Health Visiting (1993) *The Council's Position Concerning a Period of Support and Preceptorship. Registrar's letter 1/1193.* London: UKCC.

United Kingdom Central Council for Nursing, Midwifery and Health Visiting (1999) *Fitness for Practice: The UKCC Commission for Nursing and Midwifery Education.* London: UKCC.

USHistory.org (2010) *The Declaration of Independence.* Available from: www.ushistory.org/declaration/document/.

Vaarito, H and Leino-Kilpi, H (2005) Nursing advocacy – a review of the empirical research 1990–2003. *International Journal of Nursing Studies*, 42 (6): 705–14.

Vivar, CG (2006) Putting conflict management into practice: a nursing case study. *Journal of Nursing Management*, 14: 201–6.

Wenger, E (1998) *Communities of Practice: Learning, Meaning, and Identity.* Cambridge: Cambridge University Press.

Westbrook, J, Woods, A, Rob, M, Dunsmuir, T and Day, R (2010) Association of interruptions with an increased risk and severity of medication administration errors. *Archives of Internal Medicine*, 170 (8): 683–90.

Willis, L and Daisley, J (1995) *The Assertive Trainer: A Practical Handbook for Trainers and Running Assertiveness Courses.* Maidenhead: McGraw-Hill.

Wilson, J (1999) Applying Clinical Risk Modification in Practice, in Wilson, J and Tingle, J (eds) *Clinical Risk Modification.* Edinburgh: Butterworth-Heinemann.

Wilson, J and Tingle, J (1999a) Introduction to clinical risk management and modification, in Wilson, J and Tingle, J (eds) *Clinical Risk Modification.* Edinburgh: Butterworth-Heinemann.

Wilson, J and Tingle, J (1999b) Conclusion and the way forward, in Wilson, J and Tingle, J (1999) *Clinical Risk Modification.* Edinburgh: Butterworth-Heinemann.

Xyrichis, A and Ream, E (2007) Teamwork: a concept analysis. *Journal of Advanced Nursing*, 61(2): 232–41.

Zimmerman, B and Martinez-Ponns, M (1988) Construct validation of a strategy model of student-regulated learning. *Journal of Educational Psychology*, 80: 284–90.

Zororodi, M and Foley, B (2009) The nature of advocacy vs paternalism in nursing: clarifying the 'thin line'. *Journal of Advanced Nursing*, 65 (8): 1746–52.

Index

Note: Page number in italics refers to figures, illustrations, and tables.